medical readings
on
vision, speech and hearing

medical readings
on
vision, speech and hearing

oliver e. byrd, stanford university
thomas r. byrd, de anza college

boyd & fraser publishing company
san francisco, california

This book is in the
BOYD & FRASER MEDICAL READINGS SERIES

Library of Congress Catalog Number: 70-157806

ISBN: 0–87835–027–6

1 2 3 · 3 2 1

preface

Man's vision and hearing are his most important resources for the acquisition of knowledge. Man's speech represents his greatest talent for expression of understandings and exchange of ideas. Both in the individual and in a society, the development of speech precedes the capacity to express thoughts in writing.

Vision, speech and hearing are fundamental prerequisites to communication between individuals and societies. Without these resources mankind as we know it would forever remain in a primitive animal existence.

Under normal conditions each person has genetic assurance that he will be born with the capacity for vision, speech and hearing, but many destructive forces can alter this normal expectancy and may impair or destroy it. It is a matter of great concern to the welfare of the individual to possess and to defend his capacities for full communication with others.

Poor heredity, excessive light, injuries, infections, poor nutrition, drugs, allergies and broken blood vessels may impair or destroy vision. Damage to the embryo, brain injury, mental retardation and psychological tensions may impair speech. Noise, infections, heredity, drugs, allergies and injuries are some of the forces that may cause loss of hearing. The individual and society as a whole need to overcome these destructive influences through education, research, detection and treatment.

Some of these condensed and simplified medical readings have been previously published. The authors want to thank the Stanford University Press for its permission to include them in this volume.

O.E.B.
T.R.B.

contents

part 2: speech

15   speech disorders   93

part 3: hearing

16   hearing losses and deafness   111

part 1: vision

1

vision

Vision depends not only upon the reception of light waves, but also upon their proper refraction, transmission into nerve impulses, conduction into the brain, proper interpretation and storage therein for recall as needed. Anything that disturbs this biochemical and anatomical process must of necessity result in impaired vision or blindness. Vision is not a simple process; it is a highly complex one that is subject to damage from beginning to end of the visual pathways.

the physiology of vision

Senders, Virginia L. "The Physiological Basis of Visual Acuity," Psychological Bulletin, 45: 465–90 (No. 6), November 1948.

Virginia L. Senders, of Wellesley College, discusses the theories of the physiological basis of vision. Perhaps the most promising explanation of vision is the theory advocated by Marshall and Talbot. Although not completely substantiated by experimental evidence, this theory maintains that reception of light by the retina of the eye is only the first step in vision and that ultimately impulses received by the brain determine the extent of vision.

These investigators suggest seven mechanisms which are related to events that occur in the retina, the optic tract (nerve pathways for vision) and the brain. These seven mechanisms involve diffraction by the pupil, distribution of light intensities to separate receptors, overlapping between nerve pathways, recovery cycles after stimulation of nerve tissue by light, multiplication of the visual pathway, thresholds (possibly photochemical in nature), and the range of nervous activity in terms of impulses delivered to the brain.

visual development

Editorial. "New Look at Refractive Errors," British Medical Journal, 1063–64 (No. 5284), April 14, 1962.

It is well known that at birth the eye is small in all dimensions, but it may come as a surprise to learn that within the first three years of life rapid and extensive growth brings the globe almost up to adult size and functional power.

A second and much slower ocular development takes place between the ages of three and 13. After 13, there is normally little or no change in the refraction of the eye or in the components responsible for it for some years. Changes do take place but in the majority of cases tend to be compensated for, so that there is little change in the refraction of the eye.

Thus an increase of one millimeter in the length of the eyeball, which is normally found at this time and should tend toward myopia (near-sightedness), is almost always offset by a flattening of the cornea and of the lens, which causes a tendency toward far-sightedness. Even in eyes showing marked elongation of two or three millimeters it is only when the mechanism of compensation breaks down that the child becomes near-sighted or experiences a marked reduction in far-sightedness.

Errors in refraction must therefore be explained as a partial failure of coordination of development rather than in bare anatomical terms. The eye appears to be independent in its development from the rate of bodily growth, and neither puberty nor menstruation appear to influence eye development.

lifelong care of the eyes

Post, Lawrence T. "Lifelong Care of the Eyes," Journal of the American Medical Association, 119: 921–23 (No. 12), July 18, 1942.

Lawrence T. Post, M.D., of St. Louis, believes that the care of the eyes begins before conception, since certain types of eye disorders are hereditary in nature and can be controlled only by the careful selection of a marriage partner. For example, two people with extreme nearsightedness should not marry each other but each should choose a mate with normal vision.

Proper prenatal care for the mother is also essential if the newborn child is to be adequately nourished. Proper medical care at the time of birth is also necessary if eye infections (as from gonorrhea) at this time are to be prevented. Infants must also be protected from trachoma if the possibility of blindness is to be averted. In some countries, as in Egypt in 1942, trachoma was found in almost every native child before the age of one year. Trachoma is a disease of insanitation (apparently caused by a virus) but can be controlled by education of adults and the use of the sulfonamide drugs in children.

The vision of children should be tested between the third and fourth years of life. A thorough examination, under cyclopegia (paralysis of the ciliary muscles), should be made at about the start of the second grade in school. A thorough examination should be made earlier if trouble is suspected. Re-examination of the eyes should be made every two years thereafter. If disease is found then examinations should be more frequent.

In early adult life eye injuries are mostly from industrial accidents. Industrial safety, improved lighting, and shorter working hours are important to eye health, but much remains to be done to give workers their greatest eye efficiency.

In middle and in old age the ophthalmologist (physician trained in the anatomy, physiology, and diseases of the eye) should be consulted more frequently. Far more brilliant lighting is needed for reading. The older person should be especially alert to discover and control degenerative diseases or poisons from infections. Exercise should be reasonable. Proper nutrition is important to eye health. The vitamins may be of particular value. The application of heat to the eyes in the form of hot packs, infrared rays, and diathermy may have some value in improving circulation of the blood to the eyes.

vision in the elderly

Moffatt, P. McG. "Disorders of Vision in the Elderly," The Practitioner, 190: 605–10 (No. 1139), May 1963.

A surgeon of Moorfields Eye Hospital in England says that to describe all the changes occurring in the eyes as the result of the aging process would require the space of a book. This article is confined mainly to those changes and disabilities commonly seen.

1 *Presbyopia.* The first indication of aging in the eye itself is diminishing ability to accommodate for near objects. The average age of onset of presbyopia is around 45 years but there are many patients who possess strong accommodative powers and retain their ability to read small print until they reach their early or mid-fifties. Glasses should not be prescribed for these more fortunate persons until they really need them. Once people begin to wear glasses for near vision it is surprising how quickly the presbyopia seems to increase and how much more difficult it is to see without the glasses. This is the effect of providing a crutch which when taken away leaves the patient worse off than before. Ultimately, however, there is no alternative to glasses. The cause of the presbyopia lies in the lens. Throughout life the lens is laying on new fibres so that those in the center become compressed to form a hard nucleus which is less responsive to the contraction of the ciliary muscle. It is not until middle age, however, that the hardening process reduces the focusing power of the eye sufficiently to cause difficulty with near vision.

2 *Senile Cataract.* Senile cataracts can be regarded mainly as an aging process in the eyeball. Strictly speaking, every opacity in the lens of the eye can be called a cataract, and there are very few people of 65 years or more who do not show something of the kind. Senile cataracts are of two main types: those beginning with spokes or wedges of opacity from the equator pointing toward the center of the lens, which is becoming cloudy. The rate at which these opacities increase is extremely variable, and ripening of a cataract may take months or years or remain stationary for long periods, but sooner or later in most cases the opacities will prevent useful vision. Because the name senile cataract implies that this is the result of aging it is necessary to point out that there are some old people in whom these gross changes do not occur. There are therefore other factors concerned. When cataract first appears there may be no noticeable subjective change in the visual acuity but later some blurring is complained of and occasionally monocular double vision may occur. As the opacities increase in size, number and density, visual acuity diminishes and cannot be fully corrected by any lens.

The degree of failure of vision and how much it interferes with work or other pursuits largely determine the decision when to operate and remove the cataract. Nowadays it is no longer necessary to wait until the cataract is 'ripe.' The intracapsular method of extraction calls for removing the lens completely in its capsule. Provided the general condition of the patient is healthy and the eye is otherwise normal, removal of cataract is a safe and sight-restoring operation.

3 *Glaucoma.* Glaucoma, though very much a disease having a genetic determination, is nevertheless a disease of advancing years. Many more cases are seen in the second half of life than in the first half. Surveys show that approximately 2 per cent of patients over 40 years of age attending for routine testing for glasses and examination of the eyes, and never having had any previous eye disease, are in fact suffering from early glaucoma. The early diagnosis of glaucoma is a matter of profound importance if deterioration of vision and blindness are to be averted. Early symptoms suggesting the diagnosis are periodic aching of the eyes and blurring of vision after prolonged reading and sewing, failing accommodation and deficient dark adaptations, as when going into a cinema, and the occasional seeing of colored halos around naked lights. Examination of the tension by the digital method is notoriously unreliable. It must be ascertained by measurement with a tonometer. The treatment is to maintain an adequate outflow of aqueous to ensure a normal intra-ocular tension. This may be done by miotics for a time or by a filtering operation. This operation will provide a channel through which aqueous fluid will filter and become absorbed into the conjunctival veins and thus maintain the intra-ocular pressure at the normal level.

4 *Senile Macular Degeneration.* As its name implies, senile macular degeneration is a disease of old age but is influenced by genetic factors, as well as by pathological changes elsewhere. The macular changes are produced by disease of the choroidal capillary vessels which become thickened and incapable of providing adequate nourishment for the retina. Exudates and hemorrhages may occur in the choroid from the diseased capillaries and these seep into the retina and organize into a plaque of yellowish-white tissue. The retina in this area becomes blind. The patient complains of the vision being uneven or patchy and experiences increasing difficulty in reading until eventually the central vision is lost and reading becomes impossible. It may be some considerable time before this stage is reached, however, and a visual aid in the form of a magnifying device, with or without means of illuminating the print, may be of great help.

5 *Detachment of the Retina.* The subjective phenomenon of seeing flashes of light for which no cause can be found may be the result of mechanical stresses to the retina. The incidence of detached retina not caused by trauma increases with age and the inference is that the aged eye has undergone changes.

6 *Malignant Melanoma of the Choroid.* This is the one primary growth which occurs in the eye in middle and later life with any degree of frequency. The patient may seek advice on account of a shadow before the eye or because the sight in the affected eye is blurred or the growth may be discovered during a routine examination for glasses. Treatment is removal of the eye.

7 *Cardiovascular diseases.* Systemic diseases affecting the eyes which tend to occur in later life are mainly cardiovascular and affect the eyes by inducing changes in the retinal vessels. Vision is affected by leakage of plasma and cells through the diseased vessel walls, by obstruction of the retinal arterioles and venules with the formation of multiple hemorrhages into the retina, even extending into the vitreous, patches of exudates in the retina and swelling of the optic nerve head. Atheromatous changes in the walls of the central retinal artery and vein may lead to their occlusion with sudden loss of vision without pain. Occlusion of the central vein does not cause immediate total blindness but the sight is grossly and rapidly impaired down to being able only to see a hand moving in front of the eye. This may last for a few days but is eventually lost. No treatment is likely to be beneficial and the use of anticoagulants has proved disappointing. Secondary glaucoma occurs in about 25 per cent of cases within three months.

8 *Diabetes mellitus.* The retinal changes from diabetes do not appear until the disease has been present for some fifteen or more years. The changes take place primarily in the blood vessels. The trend is always towards further loss of sight, though useful vision may remain for a number of years. There is as yet no satisfactory treatment. Prophylaxis in maintaining the blood chemistry as near normal as possible offers the best solution.

education versus blindness

O'Rourke, James. "Education to Combat Blindness," Eye, Ear, Nose and Throat Monthly, 44: 47–50 (No. 5), May 1965.

The Medical Director of the Ophthalmology Division of the Georgetown Medical Center in Washington, D.C. says that despite a great deal of scientific knowledge regarding the causes of blindness the problem continues to grow.

One reason for the lack of sufficient progress in the struggle against blindness is that scientific knowledge has increased in separate fields without sufficient relationship to other information. Research biologists, for example, have had little opportunity to see blindness at first hand and know very little about the problems of rehabilitating the blind patient.

The basic sciences, the social sciences, and the clinical sciences are all related to certain aspects of the blindness problem. The basic sciences are concerned with fundamental research on vision and optics, the social sciences work on problems of screening, public education, and help for the blind. The clinical sciences are concerned with patient education and patient care. The isolation of these vision–related sciences calls for a new educational approach in which all vision-oriented scientists and professionals work together and understand the contributions and needs of the others.

The problem of visual impairment is unique, according to Dr. O'Rourke. It has clearly not yielded to traditional methods of education and organization. The present approach isolates and scatters the important professional workers and prevents full progress against blindness. Better methods of education and patient care are needed.

2

hereditary visual disorders

Diabetes and glaucoma, both of which are hereditary in their origins, are already the two leading causes of blindness in the United States. In a sense all parts of the body are determined by genetic influences. Hence it should be no surprise that some eye disorders may be hereditary in origin. An important part of the preservation of vision is genetic counseling of young people. Only by this procedure can it be expected that the hreditary disorders of vision can be kept under reasonable control.

hereditary eye diseases

Manchester, P. Thomas, Jr. "Advising Patients with Hereditary Eye Disease," American Journal of Ophthalmology, 40: 412-17 (No. 3), September 1955.

P. Thomas Manchester, Jr., M.D., of Atlanta, Georgia, observes that hereditary features have been reported in connection with every part of the eye.

Glaucoma and cataracts are practically always inherited as dominant traits. A trait is dominant when one of the parents is affected and 50 per cent of the children are affected, although normal members of the family have all normal children.

Sometimes there will occur the confusing feature of glaucoma being transmitted by a person with seemingly normal eyes. This is an instance of what is called "irregular dominance." It may represent an effect of environment upon heredity. Perhaps the patient has lived a protected life free from emotional injury, and this has allowed him the privilege of normal eyes even though he does have a tendency to glaucoma. One practical value in recognizing hereditary glaucoma lies in the fact that seemingly normal members of such a family must be followed very carefully.

Retinoblastoma is a dominant eye disease which merits some discussion. Usually children with retinoblastoma are brought to the ophthalmologist by parents who have perfectly normal eyes. Since retinoblastoma is dominant and neither of the parents has the disease, it can be assumed that they do not carry the gene for this disorder and their affected child must represent an example of mutation. Their other children should be normal, since neither of these parents is a carrier of retinoblastoma.

When a person does have retinoblastoma there is an entirely different genetic problem if he survives the disease. Such a parent should emphatically not have children, because theoretically each of his offspring will have a 50-50 chance of getting retinoblastoma. Actually, those cases which are on record show an incidence even higher than has been calculated.

Cataracts of many types have been known to show a dominant hereditary tendency. However, most cases of cataract are merely sporadic and are not in any way hereditary.

Recessive and sex-linked hereditary eye disorders are more difficult to uncover and it may be necessary to study two or three generations before the type of inheritance that is involved will be revealed.

blindness from diabetes

Field, Richard A. "Prevention of Diabetic Retinopathy," Nebraska State Medical Journal, 54: 581–585 (No. 9), September 1969.

A Professor of Medicine of the Jefferson Medical College in Philadelphia observes that two advances in medicine have, oddly enough, increased the amount of blindness from diabetes.

The discovery of insulin in 1922 extended the life of diabetic children from their previous 4 or 5 years of life expectancy to at least several decades longer. The discovery of antibiotics allowed diabetic persons to survive gangrene and other serious infections that would formerly have taken their lives. By surviving longer, the diabetic increases his chances of suffering from blindness, because the retina (which contains the light–receptor cells) of the diabetic person is more susceptible to damage than is that of the person who does not have this disease.

Dr. Field predicts that within 10 years diabetes will supplant glaucoma as the leading cause of blindness in the United States. After a person has had diabetes for 20 years there is a 50 per cent chance that his vision will have been affected. After 30 years of diabetes about 95 per cent of those afflicted will show evidence of damage to vision. There is no certain way to prevent diabetic damage to the retina at the present time.

Despite preliminary reports of the values of low–fat diets, anti-cholesterol compounds, anabolic steroids, Vitamin B_{12} and other vitamins, thyroxine, estrogens, salicylates, nicotinic acid, vasodilators and other drugs and hormones, no positive proof of their value has yet been forthcoming. Other approaches to prevention of diabetic blindness also remain unproven. Effective dietary and drug control of high blood pressure in the diabetic does seem to improve his chances of retaining vision over a longer period of time. Each year, the diabetic should have a thorough eye examination through dilated pupils. Low fat diets and anti-cholesterol agents appear to be advisable. As soon as damage to the retina is observed by the eye specialist, photocoagulation is advised by Dr. Field. Photocoagulation involves the use of beams of light, such as from the laser, to coagulate, seal or destroy abnormal tissues or formations from the blood vessels that underlie the retina. However, small areas of blindness are produced by this treatment, so it has its limitations, even though it may preserve larger areas of sight.

Within 20 years, Dr. Field predicts that a truly effective treatment to prevent blindness in the diabetic will be forthcoming.

eye problems in diabetes

Statti, Louis W. "Ophthalmic Problems in Diabetes," Pennsylvania Medical Journal, 59: 331–333 (No. 3), March 1956.

Louis W. Statti, M.D., of Pittsburgh, Pennsylvania, says that rapid eye changes may be the first subjective sign of diabetes. He contends that sudden changes in refractive errors should make one very suspicious of diabetes. Sudden changes from nearsightedness to farsightedness or vice versa may be attributed to the entering of fluid into the lens of the eye. Under treatment the condition is reversed with the fluid being drained from the lens so that farsightedness may develop. Regardless of cause, sudden changes in refractive errors of vision call for a blood sugar examination or at least a urinalysis.

Ocular paralysis may also occur and double vision may be the first symptom. Recovery, even with treatment, is slow and usually takes about three months. New vessels may form on the surface of the iris, a serious complication with a poor outlook for the future, both for vision and for retention of the globe.

The largest group of visual complications in diabetes involves the retina. Changes in the retina are directly related to the duration of diabetes rather than to its severity. Changes are usually found in both eyes, without any sign of swelling. There is no treatment for diabetic retinitis aside from the treatment of diabetes itself. Proper dietary control and insulin regulation is the only effective treatment. The value of other measures is problematical.

heredity and glaucoma

Posner, Adolph, and Abraham Schlossman. "Role of Inheritance in Glaucoma," Archives of Ophthalmology, 41: 125–50 (No. 2), February 1949.

Drs. Posner and Schlossman, of New York, report a study of 373 patients who had glaucoma. This disease of the eye occurs in about 1 or 2 per cent of the general population, at most.

The authors conclude that heredity plays a role in the development of glaucoma. Fifty-one, or 13.7 per cent, of the 373 unselected cases showed familial tendencies.

All the pedigrees studied showed a dominant heredity, except for one, in which it was recessive. There are three main types of heredity: dominant, recessive, and sex-linked. In dominant heredity, it is necessary for only one pair of genes to carry the defect in order for the latter to become manifest. If a person who has a dominant defect marries a normal person, 50 per cent of the progeny, statistically speaking, will inherit the defect.

In recessive heredity, the trait or disease does not become manifest unless both genes carry the defect. Thus, many persons in the general population may carry the recessive gene for generations; yet the disease may become manifest only if one of these persons marries another person who carries the same gene.

The genetic approach may be an aid in the early recognition of glaucoma and in the study of the preclinical and mild phases of the disease, according to these investigators.

color blindness

Chapanis, Alphonse. "Color Blindness," Scientific American, 184: 48–53 (No. 3), March 1951.

Alphonse Chapanis, of The Johns Hopkins University, says that color blindness is relatively commonplace and may be more important than is generally realized. About one person in twenty-five is color blind, and the defect is likely to influence everyday living in many ways.

On the night of July 5, 1875, the steamship *Isaac Belle*, of Norfolk, Virginia, collided with a tug, with the resultant loss of ten lives, because of confusion about the light signals that had been given. The captain of the tug insisted that he had seen a red light and had acted accordingly, although the steamship had been showing a green light. It was not until four years later that it was discovered that the captain was so color blind that he could scarcely distinguish red from green at a distance of three feet. The mystery of the crashing of the two vessels was thus explained.

In another instance a house painter had to repaint half a house because the color he had used on one side did not match that used on the other side.

This disorder is probably as old as man, and it has been referred to in various ancient writings. Some cultural groups have less color blindness than others. A recent study of more than 600 male Fijian natives disclosed that only five were color blind. This incidence of less than 1 per cent is far smaller than that among civilized European peoples, where color blindness among males runs from 7 to 8 per cent.

There are several different varieties of color blindness, and each kind of defect may occur in varying degrees. Only about 100 cases of total color blindness have been found in the whole history of visual science. By far the most common kind of color blindness is two-color vision. Most of the people afflicted with this disorder confuse reds, greens, and yellows, and are unable to distinguish clearly between bluish-greens, blues, and violets.

There is a popular myth that a color-blind person can detect camouflage more easily than one with normal vision. This is not true. One story illustrating this myth concerns a crew of eight men in a bomber. While they were flying across the southern tip of England, one of the crew members was supposed to have pointed out to his astonished friends a location of camouflaged gun positions, huts, hangars, and so on, that were invisible to them. Later it was revealed that the man knew where the camouflaged positions were because he had helped hide them originally. The fact that he was color blind led to the mistaken concept that people with this defect could distinguish camouflage more readily.

There is no known cure or medical treatment for this condition. Most kinds of color blindness are inherited. It is a sex-linked characteristic, which means that it is associated with the sex of the children. The defect travels from father to grandsons through the daughters; thus color blindness is mainly a male defect. Color blindness is occasionally produced by damage to the eye, the optic nerves, or the visual centers of the brain.

retinoblastoma

Falls, Harold F. "Inheritance of Retinoblastoma," Journal of the American Medical Association, 133: 171-74 (No. 3), January 18, 1947.

Harold F. Falls, M.D., of Ann Arbor, Michigan, presents a study of two family groups to support the evidence that retinoblastoma is a hereditary form of cancer.

In one family the disease occurred in both eyes of identical female twins. In both, the disease was soon fatal.

In another family a diagnosis of retinoblastoma was made in a girl at the age of three and one-half years and her left eye was removed. Family investigation revealed that five of nine brothers and sisters also had retinoblastoma and that the mother had her left eye removed when she was three and one-half years old because of retinoblastoma.

Dr. Falls believes that parents who produce a child with this form of tumor should be strongly urged to stop all childbearing and that any person who survives the removal of an eye for retinoblastoma should be sterilized, although the disease is frequently fatal at an early age.

3

light and vision

It has been long known that the retina of the eye can be burned by looking at an eclipse and that intense light of the welder's arc can injure eyesight also. Now modern research indicates that the eye can be damaged by various light waves and it may be that lighting standards for schools and industry will need to be reconsidered. An inadequate amount of light impairs learning and working capacities. Eye specialists are now beginning to wonder if excessive amounts of light may have the same effects. Further research is needed on this subject.

can too much light damage the eyes?

Kuwabara, Toichiro and Robert A. Gorn. "Retinal Damage by Visible Light," Archives of Ophthalmology, 79: 69-78 (No. 1), January 1968.

Two physicians of the Howe Laboratory of Ophthalmology in the Harvard Medical School report that recent research has shown that severe damage may be done to the retina of the eye by exposure to light.

In this study more than 300 albino rats were studied at autopsy by use of the electronic microscope to determine if damage had been done to the retina after exposure of the experimental animals to 750 foot-candles of light for one hour to several weeks, at room temperature.

Damage to the eye was found to occur. In general, the retinas of the young animals were damaged more severely than those of the older ones. The back portion of the retina showed more damage than the front portion. Extremely severe damage occurred with brighter lights and higher temperatures. Monkeys and birds were also studied.

The earliest effects were detected after one hour of exposure to the bright light. After 6 to 24 hours of exposure conspicuous changes were apparent under the electron microscope. Tissues became inflamed and were swollen. Finally certain segments would separate from the other parts of the eye tissues. When placed in a dim light the animals showed a capacity to recover vision, but at a very slow rate. When the exposure to excessive light was maintained for one week, the damage to the eyes could not be reversed. The damaged cells were removed by some quick and inapparent process.

Since the animals were free to move about in their cages (so they could avoid the bright light to some extent) the investigators found it to be quite remarkable that the retina was found to be sensitive to excessive exposure to light.

Only if the exposure to excessive light was stopped in time was the damage found to be reversible.

intense light and the eyes

Noell, Werner K., Virgil S. Walker, Bok Soon Kang and Steven Berman. "Retinal Damage by Light in Rats," Investigative Ophthalmology, 5: 450-473 (No. 5), October 1966.

Four research specialists of the Department of Physiology and the Neurosensory Laboratory of the State University and School of Medicine in Buffalo, New York have reported that in experimental animals the retina of the eye can be permanently damaged by exposure to intense light.

These investigators performed light experiments on 590 rats. Each rat was exposed to light of various kinds and for different periods of time, under carefully controlled conditions. Three kinds of research procedures were used, one in which the animals were unrestrained, another in which the animals were given an anesthetic and the right eye kept open by adhesive tape, and a third procedure in which the animals were given anesthesia, the eye was taped open, and the intensity of light exposure was different than in procedure two. The temperature was also varied.

The response of the retina (containing the sight cells of the eye) was tested by electrophysiological methods after exposure to light and after prolonged exposure to light at intervals of two to seven days. After three weeks the experimental animals were destroyed and microscopic examination of the retina of the eyes was done to see if there was evidence of injury or destruction.

Permanent changes in brain–wave recordings plus microscopic observation of destructive effects on the retina showed clearly that intense light can damage the eyes of rats. High temperatures were found to increase the damage to the eyes from light. Actual cell destruction in the retina was found to occur on exposure to intense light, especially if the body temperature was high.

The purpose of the study was to discover if light can damage the retina of the eye by a mechanism other than thermal or heat injury [such as the kind that occurs in eclipse–blindness—Ed.] and this research appears to indicate that visual injury from light alone can and may occur in the rat. Whether a similar injury can occur in the human has not been established. [Eye specialists have often wondered if the glare from chrome on automobiles can damage the eyes.—Ed.]

The investigators report that it would be premature at the present time to draw definite conclusions on the mechanism responsible for the damaging effect of intense light on the retina of the eye. It is apparent from this research, however, that injury to the eye does occur in experimental animals from exposure to intense light. If similar damage occurs in humans, then the challenge of prevention is obvious.

eye injuries from rays of the sun

Schmidt, Ingeborg. "Solar Irradiance Up to 100 Kilometers," Aerospace Medicine, 33: 802–13 (No. 7), July 1962.

Ingeborg Schmidt, M.D., of the Division of Optometry of Indiana University, says it has been observed repeatedly that prolonged exposure to sunlight even at sea level affects the sensory mechanism of the eyes. It delays and reduces the process of dark adaptation and affects retinal sensitivity.

Direct observation of the sun with improperly protected eyes will result in an eclipse burn of the eye or at least an inflammation of the retina. At sea level a retinal burn can occur in a fraction of a minute, although there is no burning effect when the solar rays enter the eyes obliquely. In outer space, the retina will be burned by sunlight within a few seconds and here even an oblique entrance of solar rays would be harmful.

In outer space the electro-magnetic radiation spectrum of the sun is composed of x-rays, ultraviolet rays, visible radiation, infrared and radiowaves. The entire solar spectrum is responsible for the retinal burn. The radiation absorbed from the infrared portion of the sun's spectrum (by the iris and the lens especially), for example, reappears as heat and may cause discomfort and damage.

The eyes of the air traveller can be protected from harmful invisible radiation by making the windows of the airplane or the visor of the helmet opaque to that radiation. Protection of the eyes from visible radiation is more difficult. The use of all-dark glasses is not the solution in outer space. Glasses or visors that remain clear at low illuminations, but darken rapidly at uncomfortable or dangerous illuminations and clear up rapidly again as the higher light intensities disappear are needed. [Such glasses are available now.—Ed.]

Intense radiation from the sun may affect the outer eye, especially the outer skin of the lids, the conjunctiva and the cornea. Radiation that passes into the eye and reaches the retina can cause an eclipse burn. The total irradiance of the sun is the decisive factor. Total irradiance consists of both the direct rays from the sun and the indirect rays transmitted from the atmosphere from air molecules and diverse surfaces.

The thresholds of solar energies that are harmful to the human eye are not exactly known.

eclipse injuries in los angeles

Tower, Paul. "Eye Injury Due to Viewing Eclipse," Los Angeles Health Education Journal, 12: 5-6 (No. 57), October 1948.

Paul Tower, M.D., reports that after the eclipse of November 12, 1947, in Los Angeles, California, 32 pupils came to the Eye Department of the Yale Street Health Clinic with complaints of poor vision or black spots before the eyes.

School records showed that before the eclipse the vision of all these children had been normal. On careful eye examination a diagnosis of "solar retinitis" or "eclipse blindness" was made on all 32 students. Several layers of the delicate inner structures of the eye were found to have been injured. In some cases the damage to the inner structure took the shape of the bright ring around the dark shadow covering the sun during eclipse.

In most cases only one eye was injured, but in six children permanent burns had been suffered in both eyes.

All of the children reported that they had looked at the eclipse and that an image of the sun, encircled by a luminous corona, had remained before their eyes for some time after they had ceased looking at the eclipse, but the picture was reversed, the corona being dark and the sun being bright. Later black spots were reported as appearing before their eyes, with resultant blotting out of part of the field of vision. Seven months after the injury vision had improved in only two of the 32 children.

It was found that smoked glass, photographic film, and ordinary commercial sunglasses had not protected the eyes adequately when the eclipse was viewed through these materials.

eclipse damage in utah

Whitney, J. Fred. "Utah Views an Eclipse," The Light-Saving Review, 31: 202-04 (No. 4), Winter, 1961.

In September 1960 an article announcing a forthcoming eclipse was released to the newspapers by the Department of Physics of the University of Utah. No information was given in this release on possible damage to the eyes.

An eye physician in Salt Lake City who read this news item called attention of the medical editor of the largest daily newspaper in the state to the possibility of eye damage from looking at an eclipse. On the day of the eclipse the paper gave widespread publicity to the hazard involved.

A study conducted one month later revealed that 49 eye physicians had found 31 patients with eclipse burns of the eyes from viewing the eclipse.

The National Society for the Prevention of Blindness emphasizes that the safest way to observe an eclipse of the sun is by not looking at it.

The effect of looking at an eclipse is much the same as using a magnifying glass to burn a hole in a piece of paper with the rays of the sun.

The retina has no pain fibers to indicate that the eyes have been overexposed. Ordinary sun glasses, smoked glass, exposed photographic film or x-ray film do not protect against "eclipse blindness." Even the goggles of a welder are not completely protective.

rays that injure the eyes

Koven, A. Link. "Rays That Injure Eyes," National Safety News, 69: 22 ff. (No. 2), February 1954.

A. Link Koven, M.D., of the University of Pennsylvania Graduate Hospital, reports that, in general, one may summarize the various effects of radiant energy on the eyes as follows.

1 *Welder's flash.* Welder's flash may affect workmen using the electric arc or cutting flame of the acetylene torch. Not only may the welders themselves be affected, but spectators and other workers may also be involved.

In the more commonly seen forms of injury from this type of radiation, the patient does not stop his work. He feels no pain at the moment of exposure. The symptoms come on some six to eight hours later, when he has a painful sensation as of foreign bodies moving under the eyelids. This often prevents sleep. A very slight redness of the conjunctiva and some slight sensitivity to light are present.

Frequently the patient states that he has had a sensation such as is produced by a veil before the eyes. Some workers complain of associated intense headaches and insomnia. If the exposure has been repeated and severe, there is intense swelling and inflammation of the conjunctiva and eyelids.

It is very unusual for only one eye to be involved. The patient usually recovers completely in a few days.

2 *Sudden intense light (light stroke).* This condition may occur in workmen exposed to such bright light as that emitted by molten metals or glowing blocks of metal, or in oxyacetylene arc welders, and in furnacemen standing before electric furnaces.

The immediate reaction to this type of radiation is a "dazzled" state. This is followed by temporary loss of part of the patient's field of vision.

Some five to eight hours later the patient experiences the first sensation of pain and usually describes it as "sand under the eyelids." The conjunctiva becomes red, tears begin to flow, and the patient avoids light (which aggravates the irritation). At times there is an impression of fog or haze. The condition usually clears up completely in 12 to 24 hours.

3 *Snow blindness.* This condition, sometimes called glacial sunstroke or snow ophthalmia, is not caused by the snow itself but by infrared rays which are reflected from the snow. Skiers and mountaineers after prolonged exposure to snow may be affected. Injury may occur in overcast weather as well as in bright sunshine.

The patient usually experiences signs of eye irritation, and feels as if he has sand under his eyelids, after approximately ten hours of exposure to the sun. The conjunctiva becomes red and swollen; pain occurs in the forehead and the eyes become sensitive to light. In severe cases there may be erosions on the surface of the cornea. The patient is prevented from opening his eyes because of the violent spasms of the eyelids.

When the acute symptoms subside, the patient usually complains of a dazzled condition, a lack of sufficient illumination of objects, and of seeing black or red spots, or even a large central area of darkness.

In a few days complete recovery usually occurs.

4 *Conjunctivitis in motion picture studios from klieg lights.* Powerful arc lamps or mercury vapor lamps were formerly used to light motion picture studios. Eye problems because of this type of illumination were quite frequent. These lamps have long been replaced by improved light fixtures which have decreased the frequency of eye complaints.

Symptoms of eye damage from klieg lights would come on seven to eight hours after exposure and consisted of watering of the eyes, swelling of the eyelids, redness of the conjunctiva, and a sensation of pinpricks under the eyelids. Headaches and insomnia also occurred.

In spite of the violence of the symptoms, complete recovery was usually obtained in two or three days. In some cases, however, blurred vision and inflammation of the eyelids persisted for a period of time.

5 *Infrared radiational cataract (glass blower's cataract).* As early as 1739, Heister noted the relationship of heat to cataract. In 1930 Mackenzie noted that glass blowers and workers exposed to strong fires are subject to cataract.

Glass blower's cataract is not confined to glassworkers but is also found in other workers such as iron smelters and chainmakers, who are exposed to glowing heat at very high temperatures.

Ultraviolet rays were thought to be active in the production of heat cataract. This theory has been disproved many times, especially by the demonstration that the chief rays emitted from glowing glass are infrared. This type of cataract is caused by the action of infrared rays ranging from 7,500 to 24,000 angstrom units when exposure is extended over many years.

Prevention of this condition depends upon suitable screening devices in the form of shields or goggles.

6 *Eclipse blindness.* Eclipse blindness is due to the focusing of intense heat from infrared rays on the macula, the center of the fine visual acuity. Usually the better eye, used for gazing at the eclipse, is involved. The symptoms may not appear for several hours or a day following exposure. The patient experiences a partial loss of the visual field, with change in the shape of objects and the appearance of a red tinge to objects that are seen. In mild cases the loss of vision is transient, but in moderate and severe cases there is permanent partial loss of vision.

7 *Miner's nystagmus (dancing eyes).* By the term nystagmus is meant a condition in which the eyes involuntarily oscillate. In Great Britain and on the European continent it is an occupational disease of great importance. The cause is still indefinite. Most investigators are beginning to believe that this condition is due to inadequate illumination in mines.

8 *X-rays and gamma rays.* X-rays and gamma rays produce a variety of changes in the eye, depending upon the penetration properties. Gamma rays produce not only superficial changes but also damage to the interior of the eye, such as cataract and possibly damage the retina. The lens appears to be more susceptible to x-rays than the skin and other tissues of the body. One of the reasons is the slower rate of repair in the case of lens tissue.

9 *Beta rays.* Beta rays are derived from radioactive substances such as radium. They have a penetrating power of only three to six millimeters of tissue. The damage to the eye, skin, and other tissues tends to be superficial as in the case of a severe burn.

10 *Neutron rays.* The absence of electrical charge in neutrons gives them greater penetrability. The damage to the eye is similar to that of x-rays and gamma rays. These rays not only produce cataract but also a variety of kinds of damage to the retina of the eye. The commonest sources of neutrons at present are the cyclotron and atomic blasts. Reports of cataract among cyclotron workers and survivors of atomic bombings have brought confirming evidence of the effects of neutron rays.

fluorescent lighting

Joint Committee on Industrial Ophthalmology. "The Effect of Fluorescent Light on Vision," Journal of the American Medical Association, 128: 1229 (No. 17), August 25, 1945.

The Council on Industrial Health of the American Medical Association indicates that fluorescent lighting has been regarded by some physicians and other, nonmedical, men as possessing harmful qualities not found in other forms of artificial illumination or in daylight. Both the ultraviolet and infrared components have been suspected. The Joint Committee on Industrial Ophthalmology, after consultation with specialists in the production and use of light, hold the following opinions:

(1) The ultraviolet energy from clear, blue, summer skylight is three to four times as great per foot-candle as fluorescent light.

(2) Light from fluorescent lamps resembles daylight more closely than that from tungsten-filament lamps. This color resemblance to daylight is a desirable quality.

(3) Infrared energy found in fluorescent lighting as now manufactured produces no known physiologic effect except that due to heating. Fluorescent light generates less heat per candle power than tungsten lamps.

(4) Glare occurs in any system of lighting. Its solution rests with illuminating engineers.

(5) Individual differences occur in the level of illumination (foot-candles) required to provide a satisfactory degree of visual efficiency and eye comfort. Twenty foot-candles are essential for such critical tasks as

reading. Higher levels of illumination are desirable for prolonged seeing, for discrimination of fine details, and where low contrast prevails. These standards can be readily maintained in working places through use of properly installed fluorescent lighting.

(6) Excessive light may produce symptoms of eyestrain in susceptible individuals regardless of source. Constitutional factors should be corrected as well as the amount and kind of light.

(7) Noticeable flicker is largely eliminated in modern fluorescent installations.

Fluorescent light is not harmful to vision. It should not cause eyestrain if properly installed and used.

school lighting

Tinker, Miles A. "Basic Requirements in School Lighting," Journal of the American Medical Association, 143: 362–64 (No. 4), May 27, 1950.

Miles A. Tinker, of Minneapolis, in an article prepared at the request of the Advisory Committee on Ophthalmic Devices of the Council on Physical Medicine and Rehabilitation of the American Medical Association, says that careful analysis of the experimental data employed as a basis for recommended light intensities in the schools reveals in many instances either misinterpretation of data or invalid experimental procedures.

Examination of the available data indicates that the major gains in visual acuity have occurred by the time an illumination of 20 foot-candles is reached.

Critical levels of illumination have been determined for a number of seeing tasks. The critical level of illumination is the intensity beyond which there is no further statistically significant increase in efficiency of performance as the foot-candles become greater. The following tabulation lists some of these critical illumination levels.

Seeing Tasks	*Foot-Candles*
Reading legible print (10 point)	3 to 4
Reading and study of children	4 to 6
Arithmetical computation	Less than 9.6
Setting 6-point type by hand	20 to 22
Threading a needle	30
Reading newsprint	7
Recognizing letters in 3.5-point type	Between 15 and 50

Critical levels, of course, are not adequate levels of illumination. How much illumination must be added to the critical level to provide a margin of safety is not certain at this time. It would seem, however, that the addition of 10 to 15 foot-candles to the critical levels should be adequate in ordinary seeing situations such as reading large book type (10 to 12 point). For the more exacting visual tasks, perhaps one should add 20 to 25 foot-candles. There is no reason to conclude that more than 50 to 60 foot-candles are required for even the most exacting visual tasks of everyday life.

In regular classrooms, offices, study rooms, libraries, and the like, an intensity of anywhere between 20 and 30 foot-candles should be adequate. Where more exacting visual work is to be done, as in mechanical drawing and sewing, around 35 to 40 foot-candles will be found satisfactory. In other parts of the school building less intensity is needed. Thus, about 15 to 20 foot-candles in gymnasiums and around 10 foot-candles in auditoriums and cafeterias will be satisfactory. Not less than 5 foot-candles should be used in halls and stairways.

For best vision the brightness ratios between the central field and the surroundings should not exceed three to one. It is important that these ratios do not exceed five to one, and in no circumstances should they be greater than ten to one.

Reflection factors for various areas should approximate the following specifications: ceiling and strip of wall near ceiling, 80 to 85 per cent; rest of walls, 50 to 60; wall space between windows, including window frame, 75 to 85; doors, 30 to 40; desk and table tops, 35 to 50; and floors, 15 to 30. It should be added that there ought to be an area twenty-four to thirty inches wide of intermediate brightness surrounding dark blackboards, that is, about 25 per cent reflection factor. This could well be a tackboard.

Schools should be illuminated so that effective and comfortable vision is possible. Furthermore, the school environment should be pleasing. The intensity of light should be adequate for the various visual tasks. One cannot depend upon the recommendations of intensities given in bulletins on standard practice. Controllable glare should be eliminated, and brightness ratios within the visual field should be kept within satisfactory limits.

strenuous visual work

Simonson, Ernst. "Lab Tests for Strenuous Visual Work Disclose Significant Results," Industrial Hygiene Newsletter, 10: 4-14 (No. 5), May 1950.

Ernst Simonson, M.D., of the University of Minnesota, says that vision and visual fatigue play an important role in the working efficiency of a large number of industrial and clerical workers.

To study the effect of illumination on prolonged, strenuous, visual work, a special work test was developed reproducing essential features of inspection work on moving objects. It consisted of the recognition of very small letters mounted on a long belt passing at irregular intervals and at irregular levels through a narrow slit in front of the subject, who had to copy the letters without looking down.

The head was kept at a constant distance from the slit by a support, and the lamps were hidden in a metal box beside the head. Six subjects were seated quite comfortably in individual booths, and the only strain produced was that resulting from the visual work. This strain, however, was considerable.

Within a period of two hours the work test caused pronounced visual fatigue, probably equaling or exceeding that produced at the end of the working day in any actual occupational work involving strenuous visual effort. The performance was evaluated in terms of percentage of correctly recognized letters for the total work period of two hours, and the decrease from the first five minutes to the last five minutes of the test.

The illumination was varied in six steps between two and 300 foot-candles, which includes the practical range of illumination in the work world. There was no glare even at the 300-foot-candle extreme.

A surprisingly large proportion of visual functions did not show significant deterioration. Among them were many eye muscle functions which are commonly used by ophthalmologists to detect eye fatigue in patients.

Starting from a level of inadequate illumination of two foot-candles, the performance improved markedly up to 50 foot-candles, but changed very little at higher levels. An optimum at about 100 foot-candles was much more pronounced in the performance drop from the first to the last five minutes and was found also in some other visual functions. Noteworthy is the fact that there was no change in performance drop from 15 to 50 foot-candles.

Results also showed that color seems to be an important factor in visual work and deserves attention in further research as well as in illumination practice.

television and eyestrain

Vail, Derrick. "Television and Eye Strain," Los Angeles Health Education Journal, 13: 19 (No. 65), April 1950.

Derrick Vail, M.D., calls attention to the fact that the American Medical Association has recently published the following sensible suggestions concerning television that deserve emphasis:

(1) In general, a large screen is considered better than a small one, because it allows clearer vision in a greater distance and gives a large visual angle.

(2) A distance of ten feet or more from the screen is better than a shorter distance, provided the size of the screen in the room permits.

(3) The nearer perpendicularly the screen is viewed, the better. Too much of an angle produces distortion and makes co-ordination of the two images received by the eye difficult. It would seem better, for children especially, to have the screen at eye level.

(4) Some discretion should be used as to the time spent in viewing television, and it should not be persisted in beyond the point of fatigue or boredom.

(5) Daylight screens are considered better than ordinary ones because they are compatible with more light in the room, thus reducing contrast between the screen and surrounding objects.

(6) Although television per se does not produce eyestrain, it requires all the important components of the visual act. People with defects in convergence, accommodation, fusion, and refraction may suffer ocular discomforts sooner than others.

eye damage from the laser

Tengroth, B., B. Karlberg, T. Bergquist and T. Adelhed. "Laser Action on the Human Eye," Acta Ophthalmologica, 41: 595–603 (No. 5), 1963.

The invention of the laser has given science a means of producing a pencil of parallel rays of coherent light of a definite wavelength and extremely high intensity. The light impulse is parallel and its illumination does not diminish by distance alone. A surface illuminated by a laser will have the same brightness even if the light source is moved farther away. A system of lenses can be used to focus the laser pulse energy on a very small area. The incident energy can thus be made very large.

When light from a laser is directed toward the eye it is focused on the retina and permanent damage to vision will be the result. The retina of the eye receives serious burns even when a person is far away from the laser. Lasers are now being produced that are so powerful that even their unfocused beam will cause skin burns and damage to the anterior parts of the eye at considerable distance. In other words, laser operators as well as persons far away are exposed to some risks.

The use of the laser as a controlled coagulator in detachment of the retina, however, has proved successful and other medical uses are being studied.

lighting and health hazards

Cogan, David G. "Lighting and Health Hazards," Archives of Ophthalmology, 79: 2 (No. 1), January 1968.

A consulting editor of the *Archives of Ophthalmology* calls attention to the fact that illuminating engineers and eye specialists have had a common interest in artificial lighting, but have had different viewpoints in regard to the amount of lighting needed.

Illuminating engineers have generally pressed for more light. They have repeatedly implied that "inadequate lighting" is harmful to the eyes, even though ophthalmologists have been skeptical about the latter. Some engineers have even urged that hundreds of foot candles, and one has even suggested 1,000 foot candles of lighting, be used in public libraries, schools, and similar buildings.

Research now reveals that even moderate exposure to light causes changes in the rods and cones of the retina which are reversible. However, if light exposure is sufficiently prolonged or is intense enough the changes become irreversible and permanently damaging.

Experiments with rats have shown that exposure to a bank of lights providing 700 to 1,000 foot candles of illumination for one week causes permanent and irreversible blindness. No human experiments of this nature have been performed, nor are they likely to be conducted, since the risk of blindness might be too great. However, the animal studies do raise the question as to how much light man should be exposed to. The 20 foot candles of illumination provided in most libraries and schools, but increased to 50 foot candles in many places, seems perfectly safe, but it may not be advisable to increase the amount of light by hundreds or even thousands of foot candles.

Recovery from light exposure is a slow process. Exposure to sunlight in airplane pilots has resulted in impaired dark adaptation for at least 24 hours.

It would now seem appropriate for the eye specialists to caution the illuminating engineers against the hazards of high illumination.

4

strabismus

The newborn infant may have crossed eyes because he has little ability to fix the eyes on specific objects until about the age of five months. Later evidence of an imbalance of the muscles of the eye should cause parents to discuss the problem with the family physician or an eye specialist. Persistent strabismus may result in permanent blindness in one eye, yet it is a condition that with proper diagnosis and treatment need not cause a loss of vision. The psychological damage to the child with this condition should not be overlooked.

crossed eyes in infants

McFarland, Corley B. "Method of Management for Infants and Children with Crossed Eyes," Clinical Medicine, 59: 315–16 (No. 7), July 1952.

Corley B. McFarland, M.D., of the South Bend Clinic, Indiana, says that the newborn infant has little ability to fix the eyes on any object. Optic nerves and visual pathways are not developed until about the age of two months, and other visual mechanisms may not be developed until the age of four months.

The full development of reflex pathways for vision does not occur until about the age of five months. For these reasons it is important to realize that it is fairly common for infants in these early months to show deviations in movement of the eyes, but to show no evidence of crossed eyes at a later age.

True strabismus will persist beyond this age. Usually only one eye is involved and diminished vision in the crossed eye may be noted as time goes on.

The child with crossed eyes should be treated at about four to five months of age. Should the child be allowed to continue with a crossed eye, vision will usually be lowered to an efficiency of about 50 per cent.

strabismus

Noorden, Gunter K. von. "Strabismus," Archives of Ophthalmology, 82: 393-414 (No. 3), September 1969.

An eye specialist of The Johns Hopkins Hospital and University of Baltimore reviews the recent research on strabismus (eye-muscle imbalance, usually recognized as "cross eyes" or "wall eyes").

Movements of the eye are controlled by four subsystems that are elicited by different types of optic stimulation, have different reaction times, and may be involved separately in certain diseases of the nervous system. The vestibular system, for example, plays an important part in stabilization of the vision during movements of the head.

Many interesting case histories involving different kinds of eye-muscle imbalance have been reported in recent years. Some patients have shown a cyclic or rhythmic pattern of eye-muscle imbalance on alternate days. Surgery has succeeded in keeping the eyes straight in three-year old children with this affliction.

Dr. Noorden comments that it is encouraging to find that early visual screening of children by pediatricians is becoming more widely accepted. If muscle imbalance of the eyes is detected and treated by the age of three or four years, there is an excellent chance of correction.

The author believes that nothing should be left untried when a person loses his good eye and has to depend on his other eye in muscle imbalance. (The other eye may be partially or completely blind.) Case studies show that even in an older person who has lost his "good" eye in cases of muscle imbalance, recovery of lost vision may be possible in the other eye.

Surgical correction in intermittent muscle imbalance in early childhood may cause a loss of pre-existing vision in both eyes, to vision in one eye only. Everything possible should be done before surgery is attempted in these children, and long-term patching (blocking) of the deviated eye (with frequent checking of vision in the occluded eye) may be helpful.

Dr. Noorden believes that dyslexia (inability to read) is not caused by muscle imbalance of the eye muscles, despite common beliefs.

the problem of cross-eye

Steckler, M. I. "The Problem of Cross-Eye," Annals of Western Medicine and Surgery, 4: 196–97 (No. 4), April 1950.

Dr. M. I. Steckler, of Los Angeles, says that the parents of a cross-eyed child, in their anxiety and in a very short time, gain a wealth of misinformation. Even though proper lenses may aid in straightening the eyes, most parents are not interested in the child's being fitted for glasses. With respect to surgery, many believe that the procedure is similar to removing the involved eye, that the eye must be removed from the socket, worked on, and replaced; that the operation on the affected eye may destroy the vision; that even if the eye is straightened it may later deviate in the opposite direction. The most serious misunderstanding on the part of the parents is that they fail completely to appreciate the child's psychological problems, thinking he will outgrow the visual disorder and that no immediate medical or surgical attention is necessary. Thus the child is often neglected. Concerning these misconceptions the parents should know the following facts:

(1) In the great majority of the cases, no cause for the crossed eye can be found.

(2) Operation for correction of the crossed eye is performed on the outside muscles of the eye and has nothing to do with the internal structure of the eye, and will in no way damage the sight.

(3) Surgery on the eye is painless even after operation.

(4) Correction is purely scientific and not a hit-or-miss proposition.

The emotional torment of the squinting child can be relieved quite simply by the use of glasses, or surgical treatment, or both. This should be done as early in life as possible. If a six-month-old infant has cross-eyes and an eye examination shows that glasses will aid in correcting the defect, he should be supplied with the proper lenses without delay. Both the physician and parents should know that not one spontaneous cure of squint occurs in a hundred cases. No matter what his age, a squinting child should be examined by an eye specialist (an ophthalmologist) as soon as the defect is noted because delay may result in permanent damage. Not all children with squint need surgery, and if surgery is necessary it is not hazardous to life or sight.

5

sudden loss of vision

Sudden loss of vision does not mean that a person will be permanently blind. There are different causes of sudden blindness and, if the condition is recognized as the emergency it is and the eye specialist is consulted in time, partial or complete vision may be restored. The responsibility of the victim is to recognize that if eyesight is to be maintained he must have rapid access to professional care.

sudden decrease in central vision

ter Kuile, Reinold William. "Sudden Decrease in Central Vision," United States Naval Medical Bulletin, 45: 933-37 (No. 5), November, 1945.

Reinold William ter Kuile, of the United States Naval Medical Corps, asserts that the sudden onset of central visual blurring in one or both eyes, due to spasm of blood vessels, is an emergency that calls for prompt diagnosis and treatment.

In this type of eye disorder the patient experiences a sudden onset of central vision blurring. There is usually no pain and the eye appears to be normal externally. Of great diagnostic importance is the inability to see the blue color of a small test object of about one-fourth of an inch in diameter, although the object can be seen, if it is white, until macular degeneration occurs, after which the vision for the white object is also lost.

The underlying difficulty is that of a spasm of the blood vessels. The result is that of establishing a local deficiency of oxygen and a swelling of the eye tissues, so that nerve cells in the retina are injured or destroyed if the condition persists. Various factors such as poisons, allergy, weather conditions, injury and other influences may precipitate the vascular spasm.

If proper treatment is begun quickly the spasm may be relieved and permanent injury to the eye tissues prevented. Various vasodilators such as sodium nitrate and papaverine hydrochloride have been used with good results by the author, who reports eight cases of the disorder.

sudden loss of vision

Abrahamson, Ira A., Jr., and Ira A. Abrahamson, Sr. "Acute Emergencies of the Eye," Ohio State Medical Journal, 51: 758-62 (No. 8), August 1955.

Ira A. Abrahamson, Jr., M.D., and Ira A. Abrahamson, Sr., M.D., attending ophthalmologists of the Jewish Hospital in Cincinnati, Ohio, discuss five emergency conditions of the eye in which there is sudden loss of vision. Other acute emergencies of the eye are also indicated.

The five major emergencies in which there is sudden loss of vision are as follows:

1 *Intraocular hemorrhage.* The chief complaint of the patient who has suffered an intraocular hemorrhage is a sudden but painless loss of vision. The loss of vision may be described as a "sudden veil or reddish haze coming before the eye."

Diabetes, high blood pressure, tuberculosis, and hemophilia are the usual underlying diseases associated with this type of emergency loss of vision.

2 *Thrombosis of the central retinal vein.* The chief complaint of the patient who has suffered this complication of vision is that he has undergone a sudden but painless loss of vision over a period of about one hour. A predisposing factor in this condition is high blood pressure in a patient over the age of 50 years. The patient should be hospitalized and given the benefit of anticoagulant treatment. The late development of glaucoma can complicate this condition and require specialized treatment.

3 *Embolism of the central retinal artery.* Blocking of the central retinal artery is most apt to occur in a person with high blood pressure over the age of 50 years as well as in the presence of some cardiac or pulmonary and circulatory disease.

Sudden painless loss of vision is the only complaint of the patient. If he is not seen within the first three or four minutes, treatment is usually palliative. Massage of the eyeball and vasodilatation in the form of nitrates, nicotinic acid, or other drugs are advisable. Blindness is the usual end result of this complication.

4 *Retinal detachment.* Injury, a high degree of nearsightedness, and degeneration of the retina in older people usually precede the occurrence of a retinal detachment.

The sudden or gradual painless loss of vision and the appearance of a veil before the eye are often the presenting complaints. Some patients report that it seems as though a curtain has been dropped to obscure vision. These visual symptoms may be preceded by floating opacities or lightning flashes.

These cases should be referred immediately to an ophthalmologist for further evaluation and treatment, although the physician who first sees the patient may instill a 1 per cent solution of atropine in the eyes and may cover them with a patch.

5 *Acute optic neuritis.* The most common cause of this disease is multiple sclerosis. Other causes are toxicity from methyl alcohol, quinine, lead, salicylates, alcohol, and tobacco.

The chief complaint from the patient is the loss of central vision. The condition may occur in one or both eyes. If retrobulbar neuritis is present, the patient may complain of pain behind the eyeball which is aggravated by movement of the latter.

All of the foregoing emergency conditions should be seen by the ophthalmologist.

sudden blindness

Behrman, S. "Sudden Blindness," British Journal of Hospital Medicine, 2: 1716–1720 (No. 10), October 1969.

An eye specialist of the Moorfields Eye Hospital of London reports on a type of sudden blindness in which no abnormalities can be found after external and ophthalmoscopic examination of the eyes. The pupils, in fact, still react to light, which often arouses in the mind of the physician the thought that hysterical blindness is involved rather than the true case of the situation.

This kind of sudden blindness arises from the outer portion of the brain (cortex) or the point where the optic nerves cross (chiasma) in the transmission of visual impulses from the eyes to the brain.

A few case histories will illustrate this kind of blindness:

A man aged 24 years had recently undergone an army medical examination and his vision had been found to be normal. Shortly thereafter, however, he had a severe headache and after three days dazzling lights appeared which were followed by blindness. He was later found to have abcesses of the brain in both occipital lobes (both sides of the back of the brain).

A 65-year-old man, while eating dinner complained of a sudden, intense headache, then stood up and said that he was blind. He did not lose consciousness, but became confused. Pupil reflexes were normal. A week later he was able only to distinguish light from darkness. He died a year later and at autopsy it was found that both occipital lobes (both sides of the back of the head) contained dead tissues and an old blood clot was found.

A 25-year-old woman being treated for tuberculosis of the lungs by injection of air into the pleural cavity to collapse and rest the infected lung suddenly collapsed and complained of loss of vision. The pupils reacted to light in a normal manner. She became virtually blind, but her vision became normal again on the fourth day. An air embolus (air bubble) in the cortex was judged to be the cause of her temporary blindness.

The pituitary gland may be damaged by tumors that cause death of nearby tissue for some reason. The pituitary may become temporarily expanded and cause compression of the optic nerves or the chiasma (where the optic nerves cross).

Injury to brain tissue where nerve impulses are received concerned with vision may result in severe headache and blindness of sudden onset, although the pupils still give a normal reaction to light.

episodes of blindness and epilepsy

Kooi, Kenneth A. "Episodic Blindness as a Late Effect of Head Trauma," Neurology, 20: 569–573 (No. 6), June 1970.

A physician of the Department of Neurology, University of Michigan Medical Center in Ann Arbor reports three case studies of patients with head injuries who later experienced brief episodes of complete blindness lasting only a few seconds to several minutes. The head injuries had occurred from about 3 or 4 years to 9 years before the beginning of the attacks of blindness.

One patient had suffered a compound, depressed skull fracture when he fell 40 feet. His recovery in the hospital was satisfactory, but five years later he began to notice his vision would "go out of focus" and would be followed immediately by total blindness that lasted less than one minute. On examination it was found that his vision was 20/20 in both eyes.

A second patient, a 24-year old woman, suffered a head injury in an auto accident, was unconscious for three weeks and grossly confused for another two weeks. She needed months to get her eyes to focus again. Four years after the accident she came to the hospital with complaints that her vision "faded out" for several minutes at a time. Her vision was found to be 20/20 in one eye and 20/15 in the other. She also reported some convulsive seizures followed by weakness and confusion.

The third patient, a 16-year old boy, received a blow to the left temple area. Although he was not rendered unconscious it was necessary to operate to remove a large blood clot in the brain. After several years the patient returned with complaints of spells of blindness and poor school performance. The spells occurred several times per month.

Brain wave studies of all three patients led Dr. Kooi to reach a diagnosis of visual epilepsy that caused sudden, short loss or clouding of vision with spontaneous recovery. Electroencephalographic studies were consistent with a diagnosis of brain injury related to later onset of brief visual seizures of an epileptic nature.

6

glaucoma

Glaucoma, a leading cause of blindness, is hereditary in origin, is apt to develop slowly over a period of many years and to have no symptoms during this time. When symptoms appear, damage to the eyes may have occurred already. It is possible for the physician and eye specialist to detect glaucoma in its early stages by measurement of the fluid tension inside the eyeball. This simple test should be a routine part of the eye examination after the age of about 35, because the disorder is found predominantly in the older population.

glaucoma simplex

Bjornsson, Gudmundur. "The Primary Glaucoma in Iceland," Acta Ophthalmologica, Supplementum 91, 1-91, 1967.

An eye specialist reports that in Iceland glaucoma causes from 60 to 70 per cent of all cases of preventable blindness. In fact, it is considered that approximately 2 per cent of all adults over the age of 40 years have unrecognized glaucoma.

In order to prevent the loss of vision from glaucoma, the disease must be discovered early enough, even before the patient has any symptoms. By the time the patient has any symptoms of glaucoma, damage has already been done that can never be repaired. Since the disease is without any symptoms in the early stages it can be detected only by what is known as routine tonometry by private physicians, public health officers, or eye specialists.

The damage in glaucoma is done because of increased pressure inside the eyeball due to an increase in fluid. If this pressure is not relieved by medical or surgical measures, the retina of the eye and the optic nerve will be destroyed and blindness is the result.

The tonometer is an instrument that can be placed against the eyeball for measurement of the pressure inside the latter. It is Dr. Bjornsson's belief that all physicians and public health officers who do health surveys of the population should learn to use the tonometer for early detection of glaucoma. The search for glaucoma before any symptoms appear should be an element in public health precautions and should be a part of all screening programs for the detection of other diseases in a population.

In Iceland the great majority of all males who have glaucoma in an advanced stage are found among farmers, fishermen and unskilled workers. It is thought that chronic irritation of the eyes due to severe weather conditions such as cold, winds, and glare may be related to higher rates of glaucoma. Glaucoma among males in Iceland is about twice as frequent as among females.

As an important part of the battle against glaucoma, according to Dr. Bjornsson, is the general education of the public. Health education (on the nature of the disease and the importance of having tonometer evaluations during regular eye examinations) should be understood by everyone if the disease is to be found in its early stages. Ignorance is involved whenever blindness results from glaucoma.

two major types of glaucoma

Morris, Walter R. "Recent Advances in Glaucoma," Journal of the Kentucky Medical Association, 63: 178-180 (No. 3), March 1965.

An eye specialist at the University of Louisville School of Medicine says there are many kinds of glaucoma, but only two major types.

The first major type is called closed-angle glaucoma. In this form of eye disease the iris becomes adherent to the outflow channels through fluid leaving the eye. The breaking of this channel by the iris causes abrupt rise in fluid pressure inside the eyeball. The patient usually goes to his doctor at once because of severe pain, blurred vision and halos. The eye is red and the pupils semi-dilated. The cornea is hazy and sometimes there is nausea and vomiting. Surgical removal of a part of the iris allows the fluid to reach the outflow channels again. Prior to this surgery the pressure within the eye needs to be brought down by certain drugs.

The second type is called open-angle glaucoma. In this type of eye disease there is a gradual increase of resistance to the escape of the fluid in the outflow channels. Usually there are no symptoms with this disease until it is too late. Sometimes the patient will complain of headaches or of halos around lights. Sometimes the eye specialist can diagnose the disease by having the patient drink large amounts of water. The fluid is unable to escape from the eye rapidly. Pressure within the eye rises and the blind spot gradually increases. Sometimes the pressure within the eyeball reverts to normal by rising again. The patient can go to complete blindness without pain or other symptoms.

By measuring the fluid pressure within the eyeball the physician can diagnose glaucoma and with proper treatment blindness can be prevented or greatly delayed.

glaucoma in families

Cowan, John A. "Familial Glaucoma," Journal of the American Medical Association, 191: 86–90 (No. 7), February 15, 1965.

A physician of the Michigan Department of Health in Lansing says that glaucoma is estimated to occur in 2 per cent of all people over 40 years of age and that in the United States about 40,000 people are blind from this eye disease.

It has been suspected for a long time that heredity may be involved in glaucoma because certain families have more of the disease than other families. In this study 43 persons who were blind in one or both eyes cooperated in an investigation to discover whether or not the disorder had an undue prevalence in blood relatives.

The 41 persons blind from glaucoma were able to identify 136 relatives who cooperated in the research. In this group three times as many persons had glaucoma or borderline glaucoma than would be expected in the general population.

Exclusive of errors of refraction (for correction of which glasses would be needed), the group of relatives also revealed other eye disorders in about one-fourth of the subjects. Cataracts were reported more often than any other disease (exclusive of glaucoma).

Although Dr. Cowan is quite cautious in making interpretations from his data it does appear that glaucoma is more prevalent in some families than might be expected, thus giving some support to heredity as a factor in the production of this disease.

glaucoma

Lide, L. D., Jr. "Glaucoma and the General Practitioner," Journal of the South Carolina Medical Association, 50: 71–75 (No. 3), March 1954.

L. D. Lide, Jr., M.D., of Florence, South Carolina, says that glaucoma is one of the most common causes of blindness in this country today. It is estimated that 800,000 people have this disease and that two out of every one hundred adults over the age of forty are affected by it.

Glaucoma is present in any eye in which the pressure inside that eye is too great. Actually, glaucoma is a group of diseases which have in common the outstanding feature of elevated pressure inside the eye.

Fortunately, glaucoma is not very common in children and in young people, although it does occur at any age. The older the patient the more likely he is to have this disease. It is relatively rare before the age of 35. Whenever the liquid pressure inside the eye is too great, force is exerted in all directions. Some of the eye structures are, however, much more susceptible to damage from pressure than others. The loss of vision is due, primarily, to damage from pressure upon the optic nerve and retina.

There are two aspects to the pressure effects. First, sudden, acute, severe elevation of pressure may cause serious damage in a very short while. Here the visual loss is due to damage to the retina, probably directly from pressure on the rods and cones or the nerve fibers of the retina. Possibly also there are changes that occur indirectly from alterations in the blood supply to this part of the eye. If this pressure is not relieved in a short time, severe and permanent visual loss can occur. On the other hand, if this pressure is relieved early, there may be a return of vision to normal levels.

In acute congestive glaucoma there is a dramatic, sudden onset of the disease, with severe pain and marked loss of vision along with redness of the eye. The pain in the eye usually radiates to involve the whole side of the head. The eye is acutely congested and red and the patient may see halos around lights.

The second aspect concerning pressure inside the eye involves a longer period of time. In contrast to the dramatic onset of acute congestive glaucoma, there is a marked lack of symptoms in the early stages of chronic glaucoma. Besides elevation of tension within the eye the first sign of chronic glaucoma is usually loss of peripheral vision. At first this can only be picked up by detailed visual field studies. Central vision is usually not affected at first. As the disease progresses, side vision may be lost to the point where the patient may have only "gun barrel" vision. In time, even this island of sight may be lost.

Decision as to whether surgery will be necessary depends primarily upon the state of the ocular tension, the amount of vision that remains, whether there is progressive loss of vision, and the age of the patient.

Dr. Lide believes that all patients over the age of 40 should have a thorough eye examination at least every two years and in some cases every year, whether there are any symptoms or not. In this eye examination the use of a tonometer is essential to the diagnosis of early chronic glaucoma. Any person, especially one over the age of forty years who complains of seeing halos around lights, intermittent blurring of vision, failing vision, loss of peripheral vision, and any other vague complaints associated with seeing, should have a comprehensive eye examination to rule out glaucoma.

7

eye injuries and detached retina

Injuries to the eye in industry have been reduced by legislation for protective measures until now the accident rates are below those of the general public. Accidents in the home and on the streets and highways remain as major sources of visual injuries. The use of safety glasses is growing. These protective devices give a high level of protection against injuries to the eye, although about one-half of the general public is still wearing eye glasses that shatter into many pieces in the event of an accident.

When the retina is torn or displaced from its source of oxygen and nourishment in the tissue beneath it, the damaged parts must be found and repaired or the beginning detachment can become rapidly worse. With prompt care the retina can be reattached to prevent further dislodgment. The smaller the area of detachment the less the extent of blindness that follows. Total loss of vision in the affected eye may occur if professional care is neglected.

eye injuries

Souders, Benjamin F. "Current Thoughts on Management of Ocular Injuries," Pennsylvania Medical Journal, 58: 395-98 (No. 4), April 1955.

Benjamin F. Souders, M.D., of Reading, Pennsylvania, says that when one is confronted with an eye injury, the following questions should be considered: 1) Is the wound superficial or deep? 2) Has the globe been damaged in a manner that might affect vision? 3) What are the possible complications?

Lacerations involving the eye and the surrounding tissues constitute infrequent but demanding injuries. The principal concern regarding eyelid lacerations is restoration of the lid margin contour and preservation of the channels through which the tears pass. Only utterly dead tissue would be removed by the surgeon from such wounds. Whenever a laceration of the eyeball is seen by the physician he must search for possible damage of the eyeball, and if there is evidence of injury to this part of the eye tissues he must think of a possible foreign body in the eyeball.

Burns affecting the eye usually involve the eyelids, since rapid closure of the lids tends to spare the globe. Chemical burns comprise a true ocular emergency in that adequate care in the first few minutes following exposure can influence the outcome of the injury immeasurably.

Acid burns of the eye are not common and are usually superficial because of the surface-coagulating effect of such agents. The initial damage when the eye is examined is usually the total effect which may be expected. Treatment consists of immediate copious irrigation with any available solution, tap water if necessary. No attempt need be made to neutralize the acid. Dilution is the watchword. After the chemical agent has been completely washed from the eyes, anesthetic ointments and a mild antiseptic may be employed according to the needs of the case.

An alkaline burn of the eye presents a different problem. The initial effect may be small, but the ultimate result may become apparent only after 24 to 48 hours owing to the penetrating action of the agent with resultant denaturation of proteins of the conjunctiva and cornea. Immediate and repeated irrigation of eyes burned by an alkali must be pursued until all of the offending agent is removed. Complications must then be treated by the physician as they develop.

Lime burns deserve special attention. In addition to copious irrigation with water, it is equally important to remove all visible lime particles manually.

A contusion or concussion injury to an eye may have very little damaging effect or may completely disorganize the internal structures of the eyeball, depending upon the force of the external agent.

Obscure effects such as subluxation (partial dislocation) of the lens and retina detachment must always be borne in mind. Injuries of this type should be treated with bed rest and careful follow-up study with ophthalmoscopic, slit-lamp, and visual field examinations continued for several months to be assured of the ultimate effect of the injury and of the advisability of the return to normal activities.

Foreign bodies in the eye pose a constant problem to the eye specialist. When the foreign body penetrates the eyeball it is often difficult to find and remove. Whenever there is an eye injury due to a flying particle, the possibility of a foreign body inside the eye must be strongly suspected. Removal of the object is a technical matter and must be done by a competent ophthalmologist.

Injury to the eye from radiant energy may occur at certain wave lengths such as the long infrared, the short infrared, the visible wave bands under certain conditions, ultraviolet, beta, roentgen, gamma, and neutrons, which are the counterpart of gamma radiation released by disintegration of the atom.

The cataracts which resulted from the atomic explosions in Japan were felt to be the effect of gamma radiation and neutrons, although speculation on this point continues. The frequency was about 2 per cent in the survivors who had been within one kilometer of the center of the explosion. No such radiant injuries to the eye occurred in survivors outside this zone.

There is no prescribed treatment for radiation injury to the eye since the result is either spontaneously reversible or permanent. Prevention of this type of injury is essential.

alkali burns of the eye

Dennis, Richard H. "A Simple Procedure for Treatment of Alkali Burns of the Eye," Journal of the Maine Medical Association, 45: 32 ff. (No. 2), February 1954.

Richard H. Dennis, M.D., of Waterville, Maine, reminds us that alkali burns of the eye can cause disastrous permanent disability much greater than burns due to most other chemicals.

This is apparently because the alkali combines chemically with tissue mucoproteins in such a way as to prolong the burning action.

The aims of treatment of alkali burns should be the elimination of the toxic substance, its dilution and neutralization with whatever suitable substance we may have at our command, and prevention of secondary infection.

The first part of the course of treatment begins at the site of the accident. The eye should be copiously irrigated with whatever bland irrigating substance can be found immediately available. This is usually water.

Every alkali burn should be considered a hospital case, if possible, even if this is only for the remainder of the day on which the accident has occurred. Here the eye should also be irrigated with copious amounts of fluid. This is usually normal saline, as this is immediately available in the hospital. Anesthesia is then used in the eye and all particles of devitalized tissue as well as of alkaline substance are removed. Irrigation is carried out with normal saline every fifteen minutes for the entire first day and is then cut down to half-hour intervals during the night. The next day the irrigations can be reduced to hourly intervals. Further reduction depends upon the rapidity of the improvement of the individual burn, but after the fourth day further irrigation is of little value.

Neutralization can be carried out as soon as the patient is seen by the doctor. If nothing more than a weak acid such as household vinegar is used, in the proportion of one teaspoon to a quart of water, this will be of value. This can be carried out during the first day as a part of the irrigating solution. Neutral ammonium salts are almost always unavailable.

To prevent secondary infections which may result in subsequent scarring and adhesions, an antibiotic is used concurrently with the irrigation. Terramycin drops, aureomycin ophthalmic solution, or even sulfadiazine may be employed at hourly intervals the first day, then every two hours thereafter until the eye is well healed. It must be remembered that the concentration of the antibiotic has to be maintained at a high constant level to be of value.

The use of egg membrane, which can be easily obtained, has been suggested in very severe cases to prevent adhesions. The egg membrane is laid over the eye in such a way as to separate raw, opposing surfaces of the eye structures.

eye conservation in industry

National Safety Council. "Eye Conservation," National Safety News, 69: 81 ff (No. 3), March 1954.

The National Safety Council points out that industrial operations expose eyes to a variety of hazards. Flying objects, splashes of corrosive liquids, molten metals, dusts, and harmful rays are among the causes of eye injuries.

Damage to the eyes may result in a high degree of disability and disfigurement. The cost per injury from the standpoint of medical treatment and compensation is high, and the total cost to employers and employees is heavy.

Some eye hazards can be controlled at the source by means of enclosed processes and shields on equipment. Many eye injuries, however, are caused by flying particles in occupations considered to be nonhazardous.

For this reason, some companies require eye protection for all employees and for visitors. Many of these companies have reported substantial savings through eyes saved. Few accident-prevention activities have produced such favorable results as eye protection.

A complete program of eye conservation includes both protection against injury and correction of visual defects which reduce efficiency and increase liability to accident.

The various types of protection available for industrial protection of the eyes include the following: cup goggles, spectacles, side shields, plastic eye shields, plastic face shields, wire screen shields, filter goggles, rubber goggles, hoods, and helmets.

Cup goggles and side shields are recommended for protection against heavy impact from large particles.

Spectacles, side shields, plastic eye shields, and plastic face shields are recommended for protection from dust and small flying particles. The latter three devices are also recommended as being effective against metal sparks and spatter.

Cup goggles, plastic face shields, rubber goggles, and hoods are recommended for protection against splashing liquids or where workers must handle acids and caustics.

For protection of the eye against reflected light, heat, and glare, cup goggles, spectacles, side shields and filter goggles are recommended. Cup goggles are preferred for protection against injurious radiant energy, according to the National Bureau of Standards. Helmets are recommended, however, if there is need for a large reduction of injurious radiation.

eye injuries from battle

Hoefle, Frank B. "Initial Treatment of Eye Injuries," Archives of Ophthalmology, 79: 33–35 (No. 1), January 1968.

A physician of the Ophthalmology Service of the Naval Hospital in Oakland, California reports on the initial care of eye injuries acquired in the Vietnam war.

Nearly all eye wounds in some areas of South Viet Nam are treated immediately in fully equipped hospitals because of transportation from the battlefield by helicopter to a hospital facility. The corpsman on the battlefield simply covers the eye with gauze sponges and an elastic bandage.

The eye specialists have adequate equipment on board a hospital ship to handle the eye injury cases as soon as the helicopter arrives with the wounded men.

Two surgeons on the hospital ship check all incoming patients. If there are several injuries the patient is taken to the main operating room for proper care. If the wound is to the eye alone he is taken to the eye operating room.

The equipment available for initial care of the eye patients included magnets (for location and removal of metallic fragments), x-ray machines, ultrasound localizers, intraocular, plastic, retinal, corneal transplant, and other instrument trays.

Whenever several organ systems are involved, the general surgeons and neurosurgeons operate first as a life-saving measure. Other surgeons follow, including the eye specialists. General anesthesia is preferred, because the wounded soldier is usually too apprehensive for local anesthesia.

Of the eye wounds treated on the particular hospital ship of this report, 16 per cent involved foreign bodies that had lodged in the eyeball, 29 per cent involved similar objects that had not penetrated the eyeball but had injured other parts of the eye; 30 per cent included lacerations (tears), ruptures, and other injuries to the ocular coats of the eyeball. Eleven per cent of the eye injuries involved the eyelids. Twelve cases out of the total of 119 patients involved contusions. Burns of the eyes were rare except for minor lid injuries.

eye burns and tear gas

Hoffman, D. H. "Eye Burns Caused by Tear Gas," British Journal of Ophthalmology, 51: 265–268 (No. 4), April 1967.

A physician of the Hamburg University School of Medicine in West Germany reports from his experience of treating 50 persons with eye injuries due to tear gas that damage to vision from this source occurs only when the shots from tear gas guns are fired at close range. At long range the tear gas irritant reaches the eyes in gaseous form and such shots are not dangerous to eyesight.

It is only when the shot is fired at a distance of about 1 to 6 feet from the face of the victim that damage to the eyes may occur. In a tear gas shell the chemical (usually chloracetophenon) is sealed in the cartridge with cork or a layer of wax. When a shot is fired at close range the chemical, the charge, and the sealing substance may all enter the eyeball. Treatment therefore must be directed not only at the tear gas chemical but at removal of the solid–part infiltrations. Usually, however, most of the damage is of a chemical nature.

Various complications may follow injury from close range tear gas shots. Destruction of eye tissues, hemorrhage, damage to the optic nerve, secondary glaucoma and cataracts are some of the complications that may occur. Infections and ulcers may occur also.

Loss of vision may vary from almost perfect retention of eyesight to the other extreme of being able to perceive light only. The distance of the shot and the amount of infiltrated substances tend to determine the ultimate amount of loss of vision. When one eye only is affected, the loss of vision tends to be greater, because the distance of the shot is usually very close (so close it affects only one eye).

Little is known about tissue changes due to infiltration of the chemical. It is possible that hydrochloric acid may be set free after chloracetophenon comes in contact with protein, so that death of eye tissues by coagulation may occur.

Some countries forbid tear gas weapons. Penalties have been imposed upon foreign tourists who have taken gas pistols to England. In West Germany the dangerous close-range shots that caused damage to vision were not done by the police, but mainly by antisocial, imprudent and careless persons. In West Germany there are no uniform laws on the subject. Each state has its own ruling.

blindness from carbon tetrachloride

Smith, Adelaide Ross. "Optic Atrophy Following Inhalation of Carbon Tetrachloride," Archives of Industrial Hygiene and Occupational Medicine, 1: 348–51 (No. 3), March 1950.

Adelaide Ross Smith, M.D., of the New York State Department of Labor, reports on blindness developing in three workers who had been exposed to the vapors of carbon tetrachloride.

The literature on the subject of carbon tetrachloride and the eyes, while meager, nevertheless appears to establish the possibility of injurious effects on the optic nerve.

The three cases of blindness following inhalation of carbon tetrachloride vapors presented here are therefore of particular interest. In the first case, general symptoms characteristic of carbon tetrachloride poisoning had definitely preceded the failure of vision. In the second case, there was a definite history of exposure preceding the onset of the impairment of vision, but no evidences of general poisoning were recorded.

All three patients were known to have been exposed to considerable amounts of carbon tetrachloride, and no other agent was discovered to account for the eye conditions.

symptoms and causes of detachment of the retina

Henry, Morriss M. "Diagnosis of Retinal Detachment," Journal of the Arkansas Medical Society, 63: 104–108 (No. 3), August 1966.

An eye specialist of Fayetteville, Arkansas reports that everyone sees occasional spots in the field of vision for one reason or another.

The sudden onset of spots and flashes of light is one of the first symptoms of a retinal tear or detachment. The patient who reports to his physician or eye doctor that he saw black spots and flashing lights could be nearing total blindness, for if a retinal tear or hole is not repaired soon after the symptoms occur there may be total loss of vision in the affected eye.

Any hemorrhage into the vitreous (glassy part of the eyeball) that the physician can observe should alert him to the possibility that his patient may be experiencing the beginning of a torn or detached retina. Hemorrhage into the eyeball causing black spots means that some disorder is present. Even a very small hemorrhage should be considered as indicative of a torn retina unless a complete eye examination proves otherwise.

Flashing lights are probably due to excessive stimulation of the retina (the inner layer or coat of the eye that contains the nerve cells that are sensitive to light) because of a shrinking vitreous. Although a shrinking vitreous is a part of the normal aging process, it may become attached to the retina, possibly as the result of an injury. As the vitreous shrinks it may pull a hole in the retina.

Many patients will date the onset of their retinal detachment to a blow on the head or eye. However, most retinal detachments are not ordinarily due to a blow, but a beginning detachment may be made rapidly worse by it and the patient suddenly becomes aware of the loss of vision in his eye. If a person has had a blow to the head or eye and spots and flashes appear he should report to an eye specialist at once

All torn parts of the retina must be carefully located and repaired. If one hole is missed, a second operation or treatment will be necessary. Some patients will have more than one hole in the retina. Correction and preservation of vision demands the closing of all torn places.

Reattachment of the retina to the underlying choroid (middle coat of the eyeball that contains blood vessels that supply nutrients and oxygen to the retina) can be expected in about 80 to 90 per cent of the cases of retinal detachment if medical care is sought soon enough. If the retina is not reattached or anchored to the choroid it will continue to peel away with extensive loss of vision or total blindness.

retinal detachment

Symposium. "Should All Retinal Tears Be Repaired to Prevent Retinal Detachment?" Modern Medicine, 25: 19–23 (No. 6), March 15, 1957.

In a symposium on retinal detachment Derrick Vail, M.D., of Chicago, observed that there is no doubt that a number of people have breaks or tears in their retinas without being aware of them until detachment takes place. He believes that a history of intraocular lightning flashes and a sudden appearance of vitreous floaters should always alert the careful eye specialist to a diagnosis of a retinal break.

Once a tear of the retina is discovered, the eye should have an operation but particular care must be taken not to penetrate the retina or to treat the condition very much with diathermy.

Frederick C. Cordes, M.D., of San Francisco, says that on occasion the eye specialist sees tears of the retina that apparently remain stationary over a considerable period of time, but by far the majority of such injuries go on to evental detachment of the retina.

Dr. Cordes says that an early hole in the retina without retinal detachment can easily be sealed off with uncomplicated surgery. It may prevent an extensive retinal detachment with the complications that so frequently go with this.

Hobart A. Lerner, M.D., of Rochester, New York, says that surgery to prevent detachment in patients with retinal tears is a safe and relatively simple procedure. He is not convinced, however, that every retinal tear without detachment should be operated upon. In one group of 26 patients only five eventually developed detachment.

Charles T. Moran, M.D., of Louisville, Kentucky, on the other hand, believes that all retinal repairs should be repaired. He prefers that the physician use surface coagulation to seal off tears of this nature.

Frank A. Vesey, M.D., of Toledo, Ohio, does not wish to advocate overconservatism, but he believes that too much enthusiasm for surgery may have adverse results. Careful observation and evaluation of progress should be the key to a decision as to whether or not surgery should be used to correct a tear of the retina. He expresses uncertainty as to just how much of a role retinal tears play in the development of detachment and observes that there are reports on record of spontaneous reattachment.

detached retina in both eyes

Townquist, Ragnar. "Bilateral Retinal Detachment," Acta Ophthalmologica, 41: 126–33 (No. 2), 1963.

A member of the Department of Ophthalmology of the University of Bothenburg reports that it is unusual for retinal detachment of unknown origin to occur in both eyes simultaneously. However, there is a possibility that the second eye will be involved later.

This study concerns 633 cases of retinal detachment treated at the Eye Clinic of the Sahlgren Hospital over a period of approximately 23 years. Of the 633 cases, 98 involved both eyes. It was found that the risk of detachment in the second eye was 12.5 per cent in the group studied. The second eye was affected within six years of the damage to the first eye in half of the cases.

8

infections and eye diseases

Many different infectious diseases can cause a loss of vision. The role of syphilis, gonorrhea, and trachoma in causing blindness is well known to physicians and public health personnel. In recent years German measles has been proved to be a major source of blindness when the virus of this disorder is passed to the unborn child from infection of the mother.

Infections of the eye and its pathways to the brain must be considered as serious threats to vision.

german measles and cataracts

Siegel, Morris, Harold T. Fuerst, and William Duggan. "Rubella in Mother and Congenital Cataracts in Child," Journal of the American Medical Association, 203: 116–120 (No. 9), February 26, 1968.

Two physicians and a research associate of the State University of New York College of Medicine have examined the medical records of pregnant women who developed German measles, in order to ascertain the risk of cataract development on the part of the baby. Other congenital defects in these infants are being studied also by the group.

The doctors were able to study the outcome of German measles in the mother in terms of effects on babies from epidemics and cases that occurred over a period of eight years. Epidemics occurred during this time in 1958 and 1964. The latter epidemic was the largest that had occurred in New York City since 1935.

Data from the 1964 New York epidemic showed that the hazard of being born with cataracts of the eyes was greatest for babies when the mother had developed German measles during the first seven weeks of pregnancy. It was found that approximately 27 per cent of these babies were born with cataracts, and that none were born with this disease if the mother had developed the disease in later weeks. However, the investigators noted that four times as many babies were born with cataracts from this group than in cases of the preceding seven years. The difference suggests that an increase in virulence of German measles may have occurred in the New York epidemic, but such a possibility cannot be proven.

eye disease

Ainslie, Derek. "Ocular Therapeutics," Medicine Illustrated, 6: 319–24 (No. 7), July 1952.

Derek Ainslie, Assistant Ophthalmic Surgeon of the Middlesex Hospital, reports that the most important advances in the treatment of local diseases of the eye have been in the field of infections.

Conjunctivitis, a catarrhal infection of the conjunctiva and mucus membrane of the eye, is characterized by a discharge. Removal of the discharge by irrigation and bathing of the eye is important, regardless of the type of treatment used. Antibiotics should be reserved for the more serious cases.

The likelihood of allergic reactions from the use of antibiotics, especially penicillin, in the eye suggests that these drugs should be used only when necessary. Oxycyanide of mercury is effective against almost all of the organisms causing conjunctivitis and is to be preferred in the treatment of this disorder. A solution of 1 to 8,000 in an aqueous solution is satisfactory.

Sties generally subside following hot applications and the use of yellow oxide of mercury. In severe cases giving penicillin by mouth or by injection will bring about rapid cure.

Cortisone appears to be a nonspecific inhibitor of inflammatory reactions. It does not appear to be truly curative. Both cortisone and ACTH may be applied directly to the eye tissues in small doses, and may be injected under the conjunctiva. Cortisone appears to lower the natural resistance of the tissue to infection and should not be used where there is danger of pus infection in the eye. The drug also appears to reduce the rapidity of repair of tissues and must be used with care in the treatment of corneal ulcers.

gonorrheal eye infections of the newborn

Friendly, David S. "Gonorrhea in the Obstetric Clinic," Journal of the American Medical Association, 211: 124 (No. 1), January 5, 1970.

A physician of the Children's Hospital in Washington, D.C. reports that recent medical studies have found a high rate of infection with gonorrhea in female patients during pregnancy. Some physicians have urged that all doctors who do pelvic examinations of female patients should test for the possibility of infection.

Dr. Friendly points out that one of the most important reasons for routinely testing pregnant patients prior to the delivery of their babies is to protect the eyes of the unborn infants. The worldwide increase in gonorrhea is creating conditions that may result in an increase of blindness from this venereal disease in babies at the time of birth because of an infected mother.

At the Children's Hospital in the District of Columbia 12 cases of eye infections of newly-born babies have been diagnosed in the last 10 years, but five of these gonorrheal infections have occurred in the past 1½ years, according to Dr. Friendly. Thus, on a small scale, the anticipated rise on a worldwide scale may be occurring in this one hospital.

Without detection and treatment these gonorrheal infections of the eyes of the newborn child can be expected to cause blindness. With proper treatment vision can be safeguarded.

Dr. Friendly urges that cultures of the vaginal discharges should be taken for bacteriological study prior to childbirth and that eye medications for the newborn child should be instilled in the nursery where more time and personnel are usually available as compared to the delivery room.

Any eye discharges from the newborn infant should be looked upon with suspicion by the physician. Smears and cultures should be taken as a routine measure in such cases because discharges may indicate an infection of the eyes with gonorrhea.

syphilis as a cause of blindness

Klauder, Joseph V., George P. Meyer, and Benjamin A. Gross. "Syphilitic Primary Optic Atrophy as a Cause of Blindness; Importance of Early Diagnosis," American Journal of Syphilis, Gonorrhea and Venereal Diseases, 32: 574-86 (No. 6), November 1948.

Drs. Klauder, Meyer, and Gross, of the Wills Hospital, report a study of 397 patients who were blind because of infection with syphilis. Estimates on the amount of blindness due to syphilis in the United States range from 23,000 to 50,000 cases.

It is generally accepted that syphilitic blindness results from an inflammatory process in the optic nerve or other part of the visual pathways inside the brain.

In this study, 20 of the patients were born with a syphilitic infection and 377 acquired the disease. The average age of impaired vision was between 40 and 50 years. Eighty-two per cent of the patients studied had received no treatment of a proper nature; 31 per cent had consulted an optometrist at the time of onset of impaired vision, but had not received treatment or referred to proper medical authorities for cure of syphilis.

Abnormality of the pupils appears to be an important symptom of eye disease caused by syphilis and should lead to proper study of the patient. The disease occurs predominantly in those persons who do not know they are infected with syphilis.

On an average there was a delay of 18 months between the onset of impaired vision and the beginning of proper treatment.

trachoma

Staff. "Doctors Against Darkness," WHO Newsletter, 8: 1-2 (Nos. 8 and 9), August-September 1955.

It has been reported by the staff of the World Health Organization that southern Morocco suffers from a rigorous climate, from the "red whirlwind" (so-called because the sun seen through a cloud of locusts takes on a peculiar red glow), and from trachoma.

A number of factors of climatic and social origin combine to perpetuate trachoma in this country. Trachoma, however, is not the only danger to the eye of man in this part of the world. Seasonal epidemics of conjunctivitis occur regularly twice a year. These make the eyes more vulnerable to trachoma and to its complications.

The World Health Organization Expert Advisory Panel on Trachoma suggested that this disease could be overcome by preventing the epidemics of conjunctivitis which prepare the ground for trachoma.

In several countries, proof of the intimate association between conjunctivitis and trachoma has already been observed. In an Egyptian village, for example, 50 children were observed from birth onward; all developed trachoma by the age of one year. In every case the onset of the disease had been preceded by an attack of conjunctivitis.

An experiment in 1952 in the Skoura sector proved beyond doubt that to attack the acute conjunctivitis would bring success against trachoma. After treatment during three summers with aureomycin, about 10,000 people were either cured or on their way to recovery from trachoma. This was an unprecedented development in the history of this disease in southern Morocco.

Applications of aureomycin, oral administrations of sulfonamides, and the spraying of insecticides to kill flies that spread the conjunctivitis infections were the methods employed in a number of pilot districts. These three basic methods were applied under strict statistical control in 16 villages of one district. These studies showed that seasonal epidemics could be kept from developing by mass chemotherapy of the child population immediately before the fly-breeding seasons, thus eliminating the numerous "carriers" from which the epidemics originate.

In fighting the flies it was necessary to educate the people to avoid creating the conditions in which flies breed, although insecticides were also used. Cleanliness is now beginning to be observed by the villagers, who have also been convinced of the merits of DDT, chlordane, and fly swatters.

9

nutrition and eye health

Xerophthalmia is still a major public health problem in many parts of the world according to recent medical reports. Deficiencies of Vitamin A, proteins and other nutritional elements cause impaired vision and blindness.

Night vision is closely related to the supply of Vitamin A in the body. It is almost certain that when widespread nutritional deficiencies are found in a population, greater numbers of visual impairments will be found.

xerophthalmia

McLaren, D. S., E. Shirajian, E., Marie Tchalian, and G. Khoury. "Xerophthalmia in Jordan," American Journal of Clinical Nutrition, 17: 117-131 (No. 3), September 1965.

Two physicians and two research associates of the American University of Beirut observe that xerophthalmia is still a major public health problem in many parts of the world and that it is responsible for much of the blindness that occurs in preschool children.

The disease, which occurs from a deficiency of Vitamin A, is usually associated with some degree of protein deficiency and is frequently accompanied by other infectious diseases.

Xerophthalmia carries a considerable mortality, according to these doctors, and the fact that many of the blind preschool children do not survive into adult life causes the disease to be overlooked as an important health problem. In Jordan, one of the 12 Arab countries studied, xerophthalmia had not been recognized as a serious health problem, but in a period of about 10 months more than 300 cases of Vitamin A deficiency were reported from all parts of the country from a total population of less than two million.

Xerophthalmia is one of the most serious of all nutritional deficiency diseases. It occurs more because of a lack of knowledge of proper diets than from an actual lack of good food. In Denmark it was reported in 1925 that 24 per cent of the children with xerophthalmia died. In Indonesia reports in 1940 showed that 35 per cent died. In this study, from 56 to 64 per cent of the children with xerophthalmia with damage to the cornea and conjunctivea died, despite full medical treatment and large doses of Vitamin A. Most of the children died of associated infections and it is probably the lowered resistance to disease in children with xerophthalmia that makes it such a serious problem.

vitamin A and vision

Sheard, Charles, H. P. Wagener, and L. A. Brunsting. "Disturbances of Visual Adaptation and Their Clinical Significance," Proceedings of the Staff Meetings of the Mayo Clinic, 19: 525–36 (No. 22), November 1, 1944.

Drs. Charles Sheard, H. P. Wagener, and L. A. Brunsting of the Mayo Clinic have studied "dark adaptation," or the ability of the eye to adjust to darkness. In passing from darkened surroundings to a brightly illuminated area, light adaptation of the eyes must occur. Hence, the most adaptable eyes and those of superior quality possess tolerance for light and retinal sensitivity to darkness.

The retina contains two different types of receptors—cones and rods. The rods become increasingly predominant toward the outer edge of the eye. The ratio of rods to cones in the human retina is about 20 to 1, there being about 125,000,000 rods as compared to 6,500,000 cones. The most efficient vision under high illuminations is at the center (macula) of the retina, whereas in darkness the peripheral portions are more serviceable than the center.

Cones are concerned primarily with form and color and rods with the sense of light. Twilight or night vision is effected by the rods through their chemical content, which is called visual purple or rhodopsin.

Statistical studies based on careful tests, adequate controls, and correct standards indicate that not more than 2 per cent of the population of the United States shows abnormally high or pathologic levels of dark adaptation. However, the subclinical conditions of dietary vitamin deficiency are much more frequent than frank deficiency and are worthy of much further investigation.

The relationship between Vitamin A and dark-adaptation depends on three known facts. In the first place, Vitamin A is a part of the photosensitive pigment (or pigments perhaps) of the rods and probably also of the cones. Second, many persons whose dark adaptation thresholds are abnormal are improved in their ability to see in the dark through the administration of Vitamin A. Third, night blindness or impaired night vision can be produced in some instances by feeding a diet deficient in Vitamin A.

Recent investigations have shown that dietary deficiency of Vitamin A is not readily induced in healthy and nutritionally stable persons. When a deficiency does exist, the period of recovery, even with the administration of large doses of Vitamin A, is protracted and may require several months.

Apparently Vitamin A deficiency is not common in this country. Normal subjects placed on a diet deficient in Vitamin A in general appear to have sufficient stores in the liver to maintain Vitamin A in the blood and tissues, such as the retina, at an adequate level for many months. Theoretic calculations on the average content of Vitamin A in the liver of human beings indicate that it would take the liver from one to two years to lose its entire store of Vitamin A even if Vitamin A were not present in the diet.

Deficiency of Vitamin A may be produced because the Vitamin A in the normal diet may not be absorbed in the gastro-intestinal tract and may be excreted from the body. In conditions of malnutrition owing to diseases, such as ulcerative colitis, it is entirely possible that there may not be enough retention, absorption and utilization of Vitamin A and other essentials to maintain adequate vision.

night vision

Van de Water, Marjorie. "How to See at Night," Science News Letter, 41: 358-59 (No. 23), June 6, 1942.

Marjorie Van de Water states that we have two kinds of sight. One is to be used in the day and in the artificial sunshine of brightly lighted homes or offices and city streets. The other is used only infrequently when we need to see in dim light or the dark. These two kinds of vision are due to very different kinds of seeing organs in the eyes. The cone cells do the seeing in the daylight and the rod cells see at night.

So important is night vision for airplane spotters, pilots, sentries and certain others that the United States Navy has appointed a Night Vision Board to teach naval officers how the eyes should be used at night.

The center of your eye is blind at night. The first and perhaps hardest lesson to learn about use of your night eyes is to avoid looking straight at what you want to see. Look a little to the right, or to the left, or above, or below.

Night eyes are color blind. A colored light shining at night looks, red, green, blue, or some other color only if it is bright enough for you to see it with your daylight eyes. However, night eyes are 1,000 times as sensitive to blue light as are day eyes.

Night vision lacks the sharp vision for detail that day vision provides, but night eyes are thousands of times as sensitive as day eyes.

A night pilot who has been flying in the dark for an hour or more can see the light of a candle or the flare of a match 12 miles away, even if the light is exposed for only a thousandth of a second. If it burned continuously he could see it over 200 miles away were it not for fog, haze, smoke, and the curvature of the earth.

Night eyes can see a light only one-millionth as bright as the faintest light seen in sunlight.

Night vision is not in use immediately when you step into the dark. It takes time to adapt the eyes. At first the pupil dilates and lets in more light. Next the cones of your day vision adapt to the darkness; this takes about five minutes and then you can begin to see, but not until after much longer time when the rods adapt to the darkness can you see best at night. Flashing on a light, even for a very short time, may ruin your night vision for another half hour.

The eyes can be dark-adapted separately. One eye can be covered with a patch and be adapted to the dark when needed. Much better are the red goggles worn by Navy men on night duty. They wear these when they go into a lighted room to protect their night eyes from glare; but the best protection for night vision is darkness. Lights should be turned out at least half an hour before a person goes on duty in the dark. Then the eyes should be protected from glare.

10

drugs and vision

Damaging effects on the eyes may be produced by almost any drug when it is taken internally. Drugs may induce constriction of the blood vessels of the eye and may cause inflammation of the retina and optic nerve with reduction in vision and even total blindness. Eye tissues may be the shock organs in some allergic reactions to drugs as well as to foods or other substances. Cortisone derivatives, tobacco, alcohol and methyl alcohol are examples of other compounds that may affect vision.

It can be anticipated that the use of illegal or "street" drugs of unknown purity and unknown strength without the protection of a medical adviser will increase the hazards to vision.

visual complications from drugs

Leopold, Irving H. "Ocular Complications of Drugs," Journal of the American Medical Association, 205: 631-633 (No. 9), August 26, 1968.

The folly of people who assume that they know all about the effects of drugs is illustrated in this report by a physician from the Department of Ophthalmology of the Mount Sinai School of Medicine in New York. Dr. Leopold observes that visual complications from the use of drugs have been observed in medicine for centuries.

Undesirable and damaging effects on the eyes may be produced by almost all categories of drugs that are given internally by the physician. All manner of visual disturbances from drugs may occur, such as blurred vision, disturbed color vision, sensitivity to light, flickerings, flashes and sparks, reduction in visual acuity (the ability to see), eye muscle weakness or paralysis, degeneration of the retina and blindness, constriction of the blood vessels of the eye, inflammation of the retina and optic nerve, constriction of the visual field and so on.

[In saving the life of a patient who suffers from a disorder that can be cured or helped with a particular drug, the physician and the patient may both accept the risk that vision may be impaired in some manner or other, but the significance of Dr. Leopold's article for people considering the use of drugs is profound. If a physician cannot predict the effect of a drug in terms of complications with a particular individual, no person without medical training can safely assume that he can take any drug without the possibility of damage.—Ed.]

All parts of the eye structures may be damaged by drugs, but those parts that appear to be most vulnerable to injury are the conjunctiva, cornea, sclera, lens, retina, optic nerve and the eye muscles.

Drugs given for heart disease, for reduction of body fluids, for infections (such as the antibiotics), the tranquilizing, depressing or stimulating drugs, and many others may all produce injurious effects upon the eyes.

The physician can predict the effects of some drugs on the visual apparatus since the effects may occur within a short time, but other drugs produce damaging effects only after they have been used for a long time. Many of the effects cannot be predicted on the basis of clinical experience or animal experiments. All persons who receive drugs internally should be carefully studied in terms of possible effects upon vision, according to this eye specialist.

eye damage from corticosteroids

Braver, David A., Richard D. Richards and Thomas A. Good. "Posterior Subcapsular Cataracts in Corticosteroid-treated Children," Journal of Pediatrics, 69: 735–738 (No. 5), November 1966.

Three physicians from the Departments of Ophthalmology and Pediatrics of the University of Maryland Medical School report a study in which it was found that eight children out of 15 who had been treated for more than two years with corticosteroids had cataracts of the eyes.

In 58 children who were examined by the eye specialists no cataracts were found in those who had not been treated with corticosteroids or who had been treated with these compounds for fewer than two years. Only in prolonged treatment were the eyes damaged.

Most of the children had been placed on the drugs for certain forms of kidney disease, for rheumatoid arthritis, or for disorders of the adrenal and genital organs. The appearance of the cataracts of the eyes was not found to be associated with any particular disease, but instead with the treatment.

In three children where the treatment with corticosteroids had been discontinued, no regression or disappearance of the cataracts was found after a period of three months. The investigators conclude that if regression does occur, it must happen slowly. The cataracts can be a serious threat to vison and should not be considered lightly.

[Cortisone is a hormone of the cortex of the adrenal gland which has profound effects, including temporary relief of rheumatoid arthritis, certain allergic conditions, and other disorders. Corticosteroids represent a number of different compounds of the adrenal gland cortex, or other natural or synthetic compounds that have a similar activity. The widespread medical use of cortisone, cortisone derivatives and corticosteroids in general is often necessary in order to treat or control serious illness. Complications enumerated above, however, reflect again the need to avoid all drugs unless they have been prescribed by a physician for some definite purpose. Even under such circumstances, there may be a risk from drugs that even the physician cannot foresee.—Ed.]

eye complications from oral contraceptives

Hollwich, F. and B. Verbeck. "Side-Effects of Oral Contraceptives on the Eye," German Medical Monthly, 15: 155–159 (No. 3), March 1970.

Two German physicians of the Ophthalmic Clinic of the University of Munster report that it has been previously observed by physicians that visual complications can occur because of the use of oral contraceptives by women. Blood clots in the vessels of the retina, inflammation or swelling of the optic nerve and non-inflammatory swelling of the optic disk have been seen by eye specialists.

The authors estimate that about two million women in West Germany are using oral contraceptives. Their analysis of the German medical literature reveals that some reports have been made on the visual effects of these drugs. The most prominent features are related to damage to blood vessels of the retina or to the optic nerve.

It would appear, however, according to these two physicians, that the use of oral contraceptives by healthy women during the ages of 18 to 35 years does not cause damage to vision. The authors believe that women who suffer from high blood pressure, migraine headaches, defects of blood clotting or tendency toward edema (swelling) can expect these conditions to get worse with oral contraceptives and that they may be likely to have side effects from them that involve the circulation of the eye and the optic nerve.

The case history of a 26–year–old woman serves to illustrate the foregoing possibility. She had been taking oral contraceptives for nine months. She had suffered from migraine headaches since puberty and noticed a marked increase in headaches, with giddiness, vomiting and blurring of vision, after three months of oral contraceptives. The blurring of vision was found to be related to hemorrhages in the retina. After the patient was removed from oral contraceptives and clot–dissolving medicines were prescribed, the hemorrhages were absorbed and swelling regressed and visual acuity improved within six weeks.

The German ophthalmologists conclude that oral contraceptives should be used only by completely healthy women who have no previous history of eye disease, that they should be under regular medical supervision and should periodically abandon the use of the drugs. Any woman who has blurring of vision, vague, unexplained headaches, or attacks of migraine headaches that increase in severity and who is taking oral contraceptives should recognize that these complications can be early warning signs of imminent hemorrhage and swelling of eye tissues.

loss of vision from tobacco and alcohol

Maxwell, Hal W. "Tobacco-Alcohol (Toxic) Amblyopia," Texas State Journal of Medicine, 49: 137–40 (No. 3), March 1953.

Hal W. Maxwell, M.D., of Dallas, Texas, reports two cases in which a partial loss of central vision and other disturbances and impairments of sight occurred, apparently due to the consumption of tobacco and alcohol. The loss of vision occurred in both eyes. Both patients had difficulty seeing colored traffic lights as well as general impairment of vision.

One of the patients, a 32-year-old attorney, improved within one week after he eliminated alcohol and cut down on his tobacco, and began taking vitamins. The other patient improved within ten days.

blindness from methyl alcohol

Finegan, James F. "Nontraumatic Blindness," United States Naval Medical Bulletin, Supplement, 46: 236–67, March 1946.

Lieutenant Commander James F. Finegan, Medical Corps, United States Naval Reserve, reports on 28 cases of blindness received at the United States Naval Hospital which were due to the drinking of methyl alcohol. All of these patients came from the Pacific theater of war. With one exception all of the men gave a history of drinking some alcoholic mixture known later to contain methyl alcohol. The substance consumed was variously stated as having been "ditto" fluid, torpedo juice, carburetor alcohol, anti-freeze, and so forth.

The average age of these patients was 26 years, the youngest being 19 years and the oldest 37 years of age. All gave a typical history of sudden onset of visual loss within 48 hours after drinking the poison. All had violent gastro-intestinal disturbances also at the onset. All had an optic neuritis, which subsided, with vision improving for a few days in most cases, after which there was a gradual failure of vision again.

All of the patients had been given massive doses of Vitamin B_1 (thiamine chloride) during the acute stage of the poisoning, in an attempt to halt visual degeneration, but without success. None of the patients showed any improvement in vision.

11

psychiatric and neurological associations

Anxiety, neurotic reactions and hysteria cause fairly common disturbances of vision. Vision may become the vehicle for an expression of emotional conflict or complaint. Brain damage may cause impairment of the ability to see or to interpret what is seen. Strabismus, muscle imbalance of the eyes, may be associated with deviations in brainwave recordings.

Injuries to the brain may be a source of neuro-ocular disorders. Glaucoma has been reported as sometimes being associated with emotional upsets. Physicians and psychiatrists frequently see patients whose visual disturbances are psychiatric or neurological in origin.

vision and psychiatric disorders

Clancy, John. "Eye Complaints as Symptoms of Psychiatric Disorder," American Journal of Ophthalmology, 55: 767-73 (No. 4), April 1963.

A physician from the Department of Psychiatry, College of Medicine of the State University of Iowa calls attention to the fact that psychiatric conditions and vision are sometimes associated.

Anxiety may be linked to a conscious or unconscious form of blindness. Hysteria is a neurotic reaction and hysterical disturbances of vision are relatively common. Paralysis, anesthesia, blindness, amnesia and disorientation may be seen in combination or as isolated phenomena. Complaints of partial blindness without evidence of organic disease may be due to hysteria or to malingering. In the latter case the malingerer is deliberately trying to deceive others. The eye complaints of the malingerer tend to be unilateral and he is apt to be sulky and uncooperative, with a tendency to overplay the part. Hysterical eye symptoms are much more common than those due to malingering, but only an emotionally sick person is apt to malinger, according to Dr. Clancy.

Neurasthenia, characterized by fatigue, weakness, and body complaints, reflects a psychosomatic approach to illness. The eye may become the vehicle for an expression of emotional conflict or complaint. Visual disturbances may be symbolic representation of emotional difficulties.

Schizophrenic patients may believe that they can cast an "evil eye" upon others. Disorders of perception and hallucinations of vision are often observed in mentally ill patients. Delusions of being looked at are also commonplace in the mentally ill. About 10 per cent of depressed patients complain of trouble with their eyes.

visual perception in the brain-injured child

Frostig, Marianne. "Visual Perception in the Brain-Injured Child," American Journal of Orthopsychiatry, 33: 665-7, July 1963.

A specialist in the field of educational therapy in Los Angeles observes that the child with disturbances of visual perception may be excluded from games because he is clumsy, derided because he seems ill-mannered at the dinner table, scolded because his writing is a mere scribble, or treated with visible worry or anger by his parents because he cannot read. Such a child soon feels himself excluded and rejected. He comes to regard himself as inadequate, and his disturbed self-concept may result in aggressive or depressive reactions. His effective functioning becomes disrupted.

One of the major causes of perceptual disability in children is undoubtedly brain damage. An impressive correlation between perceptual disabilities and neurological handicaps has been shown in every study, whether it involved children with confirmed brain damage such as cerebral palsy or of children with minimal brain damage in which diagnoses were made on the basis of behavioral disturbances, learning difficulties and postural changes.

In attempting to help a child with disabilities in visual perception it is far more important to know the extent and nature of symptoms rather than their original cause. Developmental scales such as Gesell's, which are based on sensory-motor functions, are most effective for detecting in infancy the initial symptoms of developmental disturbances. They are good indicators of probable brain damage.

The various abilities of brain-damaged persons can be improved if appropriate training is instituted. An effective remedial program can be devised if perceptual difficulty is detected and its precise nature made known. No test of visual perception has been available to measure independent areas of visual perception at different age levels, but a test has now been devised that can be easily administered to groups as well as to individual children.

For more complete information on this test and for an examination of sample drawings from the test, the reader should consult the complete reference for this article, which is given above.

eye disorders and the electroencephalogram

Levinson, Julian D., Erna L. Gibbs, Manuel L. Stillerman, and Meyer A. Perlstein. "Electroencephalogram and Eye Disorders," Pediatrics, 7: 422–27 (No. 3), March 1951.

Drs. Levinson, Gibbs, Stillerman, and Perlstein, of Chicago, report a study of 1,281 children under sixteen years of age in which correlations were made between brain-wave findings and the presence of eye disorders.

In the total group of 1,281 cases, eye disorders were found in 397 instances. Strabismus, or muscle imbalance, was the most common condition noted and accounted for 73 per cent of the total eye disorders.

The study showed that 30 per cent of the children with strabismus, who otherwise appeared normal, had deviations in their brain-wave recordings, compared with less than one per cent of 180 children who were entirely normal.

In patients with eye disorders, findings suggestive of some neurological disturbance were revealed by the electroencephalograph six times more commonly in the occipital region of the brain than in all other locations combined.

On the basis of this study it would seem that children who show some neuro-ocular disorder should have a careful study with the electroencephalograph for the detection of a possible central basis for the disorder. Conversely, patients who show an occipital focus on the electroencephalogram should have a thorough eye examination to rule out visual abnormalities.

emotions and glaucoma

Sykes, C. S. "Role of Emotion in Glaucoma," Diseases of the Nervous System, 10: 104-5 (No. 4), April 1949.

C. S. Sykes, M.D., of the University of Texas Medical School, reports four cases in which emotional upsets appeared to precipitate acute attacks of glaucoma.

It was not claimed that emotion was the sole cause of the disease, for the eyes were not normal in the first place; rather, the study indicates the role emotion played as a precipitating factor.

One patient was seen after the death of her husband and after ten acute attacks of glaucoma, every one of which followed some mental upset, such as refractory conduct on the part of her son, the death of a friend, or difficulties at the office.

In the case of a forty-four-year-old woman it was revealed that her husband had suffered severe financial reverses which caused dire financial straits. She began to have spells of blurred vision shortly after she became aware of his predicament. She went along well enough for ten years, until her husband announced that he intended to sue for divorce.

In these and other cases, measurement of intraocular tension revealed a marked rise in pressure following emotional upsets, with a return to normal levels under less disturbing situations.

hysterical visual defects

McAlpine, Paul T. "Hysterical Visual Defects," War Medicine, 5: 129-32 (No. 3), March 1944.

Captain Paul T. McAlpine, of the U.S. Army Medical Corps, reports nine cases of hysterical visual defects among Army patients.

Hysterical dimness of vision in adults has been recognized since the seventeenth century. The most common symptoms are weak or painful vision and spasms of certain eye muscles. The pupils and their reactions are usually normal but abnormalities are sometimes reported.

Among the nine cases reported in this study there was marked reduction in vision, contraction of visual fields, spots in the visual field, total loss of vision in one eye, total loss of vision in both eyes, episodes of partial loss of vision, and other symptoms. All of these were psychological in origin. In at least some cases the stresses of Army life provided the precipitating factor.

12

allergy and visual disorders

As is the case with all other tissues of the body, tissues of the eye may become sensitized to pollens, food, viruses, cosmetics or other substances almost without limit. Sensitivity to pollens may result in itching, burning, redness, watering of the eyes and abnormal reactions to light. Other allergic reactions may cause swelling and inflammation that can spread to deeper eye tissues. Sometimes mixed sensitivites affect the tissues of vision and complicate the diagnosis and treatment.

stress and allergy in eye diseases

Prewitt, Leland H. "Stress and Allergy in Ophthalmology," Journal of the Iowa State Medical Society, 46: 545-48 (No. 10), October 1956.

Leland H. Prewitt, M.D., of Ottumwa, Iowa says that psychosomatic and allergic factors should be given high priority whenever one seeks to determine the cause of eye disease. Psychic and allergic injury in susceptible persons may produce organic eye changes that are just as profound as those produced by direct injury, extreme lack of oxygen, infections, altered metabolism, or other diseases.

Dr. Prewitt believes that allergic conjunctivitis is the commonest allergic eye disease. It occurs seasonally as a manifestation of hay fever and chronic allergic nasal disease, or it may occur as a vernal catarrh.

Allergic swelling of the eyelid is often a reaction associated with generalized skin disease. Acute reactions may be due to a variety of allergens, although antibiotics and drugs such as penicillin and aspirin should always be given consideration. Emotional upsets, family incompatibilities, and economic difficulties may produce generalized urticaria and swelling of the eyelids, according to Dr. Prewitt.

A variety of other disorders of the eye are described as being due to allergic factors. If the psychogenic overlay is evaluated and eliminated, the so-called drug-fast and allergic cases often respond to treatment at once. Dr. Prewitt finds it is helpful to have the patient name the feeling—such as anger, anxiety, fear, worry, jealousy, or resentment—which underlies the physical manifestation of his problem and to name specifically the person— such as husband, wife, mother-in-law, or employer—who is stimulating the emotion, and then to outline nondestructive courses of action that can be used as emotional outlets.

The physician must keep in mind, however, that one can sensitize a patient to emotional aspects by the questions he asks and by the implications he lets fall. This may lead the patient to believe that all of his difficulty is due to emotional stress, when in reality he may have other causes of the eye disease.

allergy and eye tissues

Lemoine, Albert N., Sr. "Common Manifestations of Allergy in Ophthalmology," Transactions American Academy of Ophthalmology and Otolaryngology, 58: 125-27 (No. 1), January-February 1954.

Albert N. Lemoine, Sr., M.D., of Kansas City, Missouri, states that allergy is a hypersensitivity of tissue cells to allergens. Practically every tissue cell of the body may become hypersensitive. These facts apply especially to tissue of the eyes.

The most common symptoms of allergic dermatitis of the skin of the eyelids are itching, burning, redness, and swelling in the acute phase, with a change to scaling and brown discoloration along with wrinkling of the skin in the more chronic stages.

Allergic reactions of the eyelids may be due to almost any contact substance, focus of infection, or food. Any cosmetic may be the exciting cause. There is no such thing as a nonallergic cosmetic for all people. Any medicine may be the cause in certain individuals. Many foods may precipitate or aggravate an allergy. Liquors, tobacco, and refined sugars may aggravate the allergic reaction in many persons.

The most common symptoms of allergy in the conjunctiva are itching, burning, the sensation of a foreign body, sensitivity to light, and the formation of tears. There may also be a possible superimposed bacterial infection in allergies affecting this part of the eye. With the intense itching and discharge patients are prone to rub their eyes, and the tissues may become an ideal culture medium for bacteria.

The cornea, or outer surface of the eyeball, may also reflect an allergic reaction to various substances. Dr. Lemoine states that he observed one patient who had a recurrent ulcer in the cornea every time she ate chocolate. Small ulcers that cover the whole cornea are frequently allergic in origin. They may be due either to substances with which the eye tissues come into contact or to foods.

Inflammation of the retina of the eye and optic neuritis may also be due to an allergy from infection.

13

cataracts

The causes of many cataracts have not been determined by medical science. It is likely that cataracts may be due to many different causes, such as toxic substances, nutritional deficiencies, radiation, old age, diabetes, drugs and other substances.

Cataracts can be removed by eye surgeons with benefits, but there are sometimes possible complications or disadvantages that should be considered in advance.

environmental factors in cataracts

Dhir, S. P., R. Detels, and E. R. Alexander. "The Role of Environmental Factors in Cataract, Pterygium and Trachoma," American Journal of Ophthalmology, 64: 128–135 (No. 1), July 1967.

Three physicians of the University of Washington School of Medicine in Seattle report that they believe environmental factors play a role in the cause of eye diseases.

In this study the authors report a comparison of ethnic groups in India (the Punjabis) in terms of three eye diseases with groups in British Columbia, Sacramento and the Imperial Valley in California.

Radiation from the sun is greater in the Indian areas studied than in British Columbia, and the difference paralleled the difference in the prevalence of cataract in the two areas. Also, the authors found more sunlight in the Sacramento and Imperial Valley regions of California and also more cataracts there than in British Columbia. However, they admit it is not possible to prove whether this parallel between solar radiation and cataracts is related to their cause. Experimental radiation of the lens of the eye with ultraviolet and infrared waves has produced cataracts in the laboratory. Whether this same effect is produced in a natural setting is undetermined.

With more solar radiation in Kurali, India than in British Columbia, and with an appearance of cataracts about 10 years earlier in the former area, the authors speculate that over a period of years greater exposure to radiation from the sun may cause the appearance of cataract in the eyes. Kurali has intense sunlight, little rain, and is hot, dry, and dusty most of the year. British Columbia has high rainfall, little sun, and low or moderate temperatures. Indians who have emigrated from Kurali to British Columbia show a lower prevalence of cataracts than occurs in their native country. The authors therefore speculate, but do not prove, that the environment may have an influence on the production of cataracts.

cataracts

Bellows, John G. "Lens and Vitreous," Archives of Ophthalmology, 47: 516-37(No. 4), April 1952.

John G. Bellows, M.D., of Chicago, Illinois, reports on a survey of the literature pertaining to the lens and vitreous material of the eye.

Cataracts have been reported as being due to a number of different factors, including congenital or hereditary disease, diabetes, tetany, mongolism, and endocrine disorders. Cataract may also be caused by certain toxic substances. Galactose is one substance that will cause cataract, although this is rare in human beings. Only about half a dozen cases of this type of cataract have been reported. A deficiency of carbohydrate metabolism is involved, with the liver unable to change galactose to glucose. The former accumulates in the blood and causes damage to the lens. If the condition is discovered soon enough, a diet that is free of galactose will prevent appearance of the disorder.

Some cases of cataract have been shown to be due to x-ray irradiation. Radiation in general, including that of atomic warfare, may be damaging to the lens of the eye.

Electrical accidents and exposure to heat may cause cataract. Numerous cataracts are due to changes of old age, but no single factor can be incriminated as the only cause of cataracts. The condition may be a result of many different things.

eye cataracts in older persons

Goar, Everett L. "Cataract Removal in Elderly Persons," Texas Medicine, 62: 40–41, May 1966.

A Houston, Texas physician reports that everyone who lives long enough has cataracts. Between 40 and 45, a person with normal eyes begins to use reading glasses. This is because the lens fibers are losing elasticity and can no longer mold the lens; hence, the person's power of accommodation begins to fail.

Cataract removal can be performed surgically, and many people benefit considerably by such surgery. However, the author points out that cataract removal is not always advisable for elderly persons. He believes that many people with cataracts can get along well enough without surgery. While such surgery is to the surgeon a very small event, to the patient it is often one of life's crises.

As an example, the author considers the situation of an old person whose vision is failing—who cannot, for instance, read street signs so well, and who can no longer follow the flight of a golf ball. If it is discovered that he has cataracts and an operation follows, then he has to have an operation on the second eye or wear a contact lens; otherwise he loses binocular vision.

If the eye is fitted with a contact lens, the other eye must be blurred out or the patient will see double. In this case his last situation is worse than his first. Not every patient gets along with a contact lens. If he is palsied, impatient, or neurotic, both he and the doctor may be in for a hard time.

Many nervous persons have great difficulty in adjusting to a cataract lens. It makes objects look larger and closer and restricts the field of vision. If these miseries are added to the others that accompany the aging process, they are hard to bear and should not be inflicted upon a person who can still see well enough to do everything he wants to.

The author states that he has observed many old persons with cataracts get along successfully for years until they died with the cataracts unremoved. Some of these had been told years ago that they had cataracts which should be operated on. Old people deserve a careful eye examination, individual consideration, and education on the subject before such surgery is performed.

radiation cataract

Shoch, David. "Radiation Cataract," Illinois Medical Journal, 110: 14–15 (No. 1), July 1956.

David Shoch, M.D., of the Department of Ophthalmology of Northwestern University Medical School in Chicago, says that it has long been known that radiation may produce cataract. A classic example is glassblower's cataract, which we now know is a heat-produced one due to the absorption of infrared rays by the lens of the eye.

After the explosion of the atomic bombs in Japan at the end of World War II, the whole field of ionizing radiation injury received intensive study. Along with other tissues, the eyes came under investigation. These investigations consisted chiefly of the description of the cataracts found in survivors of the Hiroshima and Nagasaki bombings. In 1949 cataracts were found in a group of our own physicists who had been inadvertently exposed to their cyclotron beams. The government immediately established a Committee on Radiation Cataracts to conduct research on this problem.

These lines of research were conducted: whether or not cataract is the result of injury by toxic products produced because of general body irradiation; whether or not there is a direct action on the cells of the lens of the eye by radiation is also being investigated.

The local effect of generalized irradiation of the body was quickly eliminated as a factor by animal research. The irradiation of rabbits with the head protected showed that no cataracts developed unless enormous dosages were used. On the other hand, a small dose close to the eyes, with the rest of the body protected, did produce cataracts.

14

eyeglasses and eye specialists

Many different kinds of eyeglasses are now available to those persons with impaired vision, but selections should be made only after professional diagnosis and advice. The hazard of self-prescription lies mostly in the possibility that postponement of professional examination may permit progression of some visual disorders to blindness.

If contact lenses are used the wearer should know about complications that may occur and about certain precautions that should be taken. As indicated in an earlier chapter, safety glasses are now recommended by the medical profession.

hazards of self-prescribed glasses

Foote, Franklin M. "Self-Prescribed Glasses, A Safety Problem," National Safety News, 69: 118–19 (No. 3), March 1954.

Franklin M. Foote, M.D., executive director of the National Association for the Prevention of Blindness, reports that forty-two states still permit a man to diagnose and prescribe for his own visual deficiencies. The hazard of this procedure is increased because some manufacturers provide equipment for these self-doctors.

Only six states have recognized the insidious danger in the self-prescribing of corrective spectacles. These states are Maine, Massachusetts, Minnesota, Kansas, New York, and Rhode Island. The lawmakers of these states have realized that over-the-counter sale of lenses intended to "correct" a person's vision may lead to accidents or physiological disturbances which the patient may not attribute to the glasses.

The greatest hazard of these ready-made corrective spectacles is that they may conceal for months the symptoms of a condition that will eventually lead to blindness and thus may keep a person away from proper treatment of a progressive sight-destroying disease until it is too late to save the vision of the individual.

All the states and the District of Columbia have laws governing the practice of eye care. These laws were enacted to protect the people. The governing bodies of the states saw the danger inherent in allowing totally untrained persons to prescribe for patients with visual deficiencies. A majority of the states, however, have created a paradox, for they have established laws to protect the individual against poor diagnosis and prescription of glasses by untrained persons but they have not provided for protection of the individual against himself.

eyeglasses

Garb, Solomon. "Eyeglasses as a Therapeutic Agent," New York State Journal of Medicine, 57: 3167–73 (No. 19), October 1, 1957.

Solomon Garb, M.D., in summarizing the discussions of eyeglasses as a therapeutic agent at a recent conference at the Cornell University Medical College and the New York Hospital, says that some commonly held notions about eyeglasses are erroneous.

Ordinary glasses correct refractive errors in vision but do not influence the progression or retardation of the error. Eyeglasses do not protect sight and may be dispensed with without the risk of affecting the basic condition.

One view expressed at the conference was that there is no such thing as eyestrain. Excessive use of the eyes may produce tiredness of the eye muscles but adequate rest restores them as it does any other tired muscle.

Contact lenses were described as being essential in some situations, but as a rule they have no advantage over spectacles. Some patients demand contact lenses for reasons of vanity. They are best tolerated by people who need them for reasons other than the wish to present a pleasing appearance.

Relatively few headaches are of ocular origin, so patients with headaches should not necessarily be referred to the eye specialist first.

Eyeglasses are of value in certain cases of extraocular muscle imbalance.

Eye exercises do not actually improve vision; they train the patient to recognize defective or blurred images.

With increasing presbyopia more illumination is needed for efficient reading, but the degree of illumination does not alter the progress of the conditon.

Glasses should not be forced on a patient who does not wish to wear them and who can manage without them.

aids for low vision

Gordon, Dan M., and Charles G. Ritter. "Low Vision Aids in Ophthalmology," New York State Journal of Medicine, 57: 3466–70 (No. 21), November 1, 1957.

Dan M. Gordon, M.D., and Charles G. Ritter, M.D., of New York City, report that during the past several years great strides have been made in the direction of supplying better visual aids for the near-blind.

Various types of devices are now available to help the patient with low vision. These include such devices as 1) high plus lenses; 2) microscopic lenses; 3) telescopic lenses; 4) contact lenses; 5) projection devices.

There are various forms of high plus lenses in use either as reading glasses, bifocals, or trifocals. Built-in or cut-in plus segments are carried on a lens which is a relatively light-weight piece of plastic or glass. High plus lenses are excellent when the patient can employ them, although unfortunately many ophthalmologists are prejudiced by training in favor of something which can be worn on the nose. High plus lenses have the disadvantage of being relatively more expensive than the average magnifier and must be tailored to the patient's specification.

Microscopic lenses usually consist of two or more plus lenses separated by an air space.

Telescopic lenses use a minus and a plus lens separated by the equivalent of their focal lengths. A conventional opera glass is the best known example of this class of lenses. Telescopic lenses are employed for distance vision for people who cannot be helped appreciably by spectacle lenses.

Contact lenses are very useful when the eye specialist is dealing with scarred corneas or with some other corneal disease which may be the chief reason for the patient's loss of vision. Contact lenses are also applicable in highly myopic (nearsighted) subjects. They are also very useful in patients who have had cataract surgery. Contact lenses are expensive, however.

Magnification devices include the hand magnifiers or magnifiers which possess built-in stands. The conventional Sherlock Holmes type of magnifier which is seen in the average store window is, as a rule, only one and one-half or two times in strength. However, various other forms of magnifying devices are now available in much greater strengths.

Projection devices are available that contain built-in projectors and screens within the single instrument. These devices can provide 12 to 25 times magnification. Only one word at a time can be seen with 25 times magnification, but with 12 times magnification several words may be seen on the screen at one time. However, even with the high types of magnification some patients learn to read quite rapidly.

No patient who is able to perceive the large target on the Snellen chart or who is able to recognize its objects should be considered as hopeless until he has been given a fair trial with the devices described. Most of these devices are available for use only in near vision. Telescopic lenses are very useful in watching movies, sports events, television, and so forth. However, because of the amount of parallax induced it is almost impossible to walk around while wearing a pair of these. The only good device today for the patient who wants to be helped for ambulatory distant vision is the conventional spectacle-type glass.

telescopic spectacles

Birge, Henry L., and Leon W. Zimmerman. "Telescopic Spectacles," Connecticut State Medical Journal, 17: 985–87 (No. 12), December 1953.

Henry L. Birge, M.D., and Leon W. Zimmerman, M.D., of Hartford, Connecticut, report that telescopic and microscopic spectacles have a larger range of usefulness than is generally appreciated. Most eye specialists have failed to show patients with sub-normal vision the possibilities of these lenses, and because of this failure both patients and the profession have suffered.

Telescopic or microscopic spectacles should be routinely offered to all people with subnormal vision. The telescopic lens should receive special consideration in the case of patients with permanently impaired vision following surgery for brain tumor, for inoperable cataracts that seriously impair vision, in cases of advanced but arrested glaucoma, extensive nearsightedness, eye defects present from birth, and a number of other visual disorders.

When a complete eye examination has revealed that subnormal vision cannot be improved by ordinary fitting of glasses or by other treatment, the telescopic test set should be used to discover whether or not vision can be improved with the telescopic spectacles. The only adverse aspect of properly fitted telescopic lenses is their cost. Many people who could benefit from these lenses do not have the resources to spend on this type of visual aid. It may be possible to overcome this objection through the use of charitable organizations.

contact lenses

Keeney, Arthur H., and H. Lyle Duerson, Jr. "Contact Lenses: Current Concepts and Local Use," Journal of the Kentucky State Medical Association, 52: 87-91 (No. 2), February 1954.

Arthur H. Keeney, M.D., and H. Lyle Duerson, Jr., of Louisville, Kentucky, report that contact lenses appear to date from 1801 when Sir Thomas Young made a crude water-filled apparatus with a lens at the end of a glass tube one-fourth inch long.

The first contact lens to be worn for any period of time was prescribed in Bonn in 1877. This lens was worn as a protective shell for twenty-one years by a patient.

Today there are four general types of contact lenses in use. The "conventional" contact lens is a molded plastic product that requires an artificial solution between the lens and cornea. This fluid factor and the blocking of atmospheric oxygen are constant limitations to its use.

Other types of contact lenses are tear-filled. These lenses have a hole to allow exchange of oxygen and tears. This is generally the most satisfactory type because the problems of artificial solutions and oxygen deprivation are eliminated. English specialists have pioneered with glass and plastic lenses of this type since the end of World War II. Other lenses depend upon looseness of fit for oxygen exchange rather than the presence of a hole.

Corneal lenses are small discs which are held in place by capillary attraction to the cornea. Approximately 60 per cent of patients for whom these lenses have been approved cannot tolerate them on the basis of mechanical or psychological problems in fitting.

Contact lenses are not suitable for all patients. They should not be used in minor refractive errors, allergy to plastic, presbyopia, hay fever, active or chronic infections of the lids or conjunctiva, emotional instability, and a number of other conditions.

The lenses may be used with advantage, however, in refractive errors of the cornea, in irregular astigmatism, in cases in which there is a difference in the size of the image in each eye, for the improvement of appearance of unsightly and shrunken eyeballs, and for various other conditions. About 80 per cent of all contact lenses are fitted for cosmetic purposes. Swimmers and participants in vigorous athletics who are dependent upon improved vision are afforded considerable safety and protection by contact lenses.

how long can contact lenses be worn safely?

Nauheim, Jack Stanley. "Corneal Ulcer Due to Prolonged Wearing of Corneal Contact Lenses," American Journal of Ophthalmology, 53: 678–81 (No. 4), April 1962.

Jack Stanley Nauheim, M.D. of Jackson Heights, New York observes that the use of contact lenses is accompanied by the risk of corneal damage. The medical literature contains a number of reports of damage to the eyes from the continuous wearing of contact lenses. Damage usually results from improperly fitting lenses or failure of the patient to exercise proper care in the handling and wearing of his lenses.

Dr. Nauheim reports the case of a 19-year-old airman who was seen in an eye clinic with complaints of pain, redness, and light sensitivity of the right eye. He had been wearing contact lenses for three to four weeks and had not removed them for fear of losing them. The left eye had suffered only superficial damage, but the right eye had a deep ulcer of the cornea which on bacteriological test was shown to be infected with both strep-tococci and staphylocci. After treatment the young man had a corneal scar two millimeters in diameter although his vision return to normal.

Dr. Nauheim emphasizes that contact lenses should always be removed at bedtime, although patients can often wear such lenses for 16 to 18 hours without trouble. Because infections may occur from a number of sources, the hands should always be cleansed with soap and water before insertion of contact lenses. At first they should not be worn for more than several hours a day with a gradual increase in the time they are worn. They should not be worn if there are certain types of infections in any part of the body, such as those of herpes simplex or those of bacterial origin. The lenses themselves should be cleaned in antiseptic solution before insertion.

complications from contact lenses

Dixon, Joseph M., Charles A. Young, Joseph A. Baldone, G. Peter Halberg, Whitney Sampson and William Stone. "Complications Associated With the Wearing of Contact Lenses," Journal of the American Medical Association, 195: 117-119 (No. 11), March 14, 1966.

Six specialists of the Association of Ophthalmology observe that the popularity of contact lenses has exceeded public knowledge of their potential hazards. These physicians report a survey in which questionnaires were mailed to eye specialists regarding complications from the wearing of contact lenses by their patients.

Of the physicians polled 1,904 responded. These doctors had seen 49,954 patients wearing contact lenses. They reported three categories of complications, in which: 1) eyes were blinded or needed to be removed; 2) eyes showed vision which had been permanently damaged; and 3) eye conditions which could be controlled and returned to normal by proper treatment.

The eye specialists report that the wearing of contact lenses is an abnormal condition which can result in serious medical complications which may require prompt medical diagnosis and treatment.

Fourteen patients became completely blind or had to have an eye removed because of the development of serious infections. One hundred fifty-seven physicians reported cases in which the eye had become permanently damaged by scars or other defects. In 7,607 patients there was some damage to the eye but there was recovery with treatment without permanent eye damage.

The eye specialists reported that the majority of people who wear contact lenses will have some degree of change of the eye tissues or some kind of medical problem associated with their use.

should near-sighted children wear glasses all the time?

Miles, Paul W. "Should the Myopic Child Wear Glasses All the Time?" American Journal of Ophthalmology, 53: 866–67 (No. 5), May 1962.

Paul W. Miles, M.D. of St. Louis, Missouri reports that ophthalmologists are in disagreement as to whether the myopic (near-sighted) child should wear corrective glasses all the time.

Dr. Miles reports a study of 10 years in which he measured the visual capacity of 28 children at about the age of eight years and regularly thereafter. None of these children wore glasses for one to four years, but later all wore glasses full time for one to six years. The rate of myopic change remained the same with or without glasses over a significant duration of time. Dr. Miles has concluded from his study that children with the usual type of myopia (near-sightedness) need not be forced to wear glasses full time.

eye specialists

Jung, F. J. "Whom Shall I Consult About My Eyes?" Journal of School Health, 17: 224–26 (No. 8), October 1947.

F. J. Jung, M.D., says there are various professional groups, differing in training and viewpoint, which are equipped to solve various problems regarding eyesight. It is often important to know what these differences are.

The most responsible work is that of the ophthalmologist. He is also known to the public as the oculist or eye-specialist, and the reason why his responsibilities are so great is that he is often relied upon to use his skill in cases where mistakes, neglect, or awkwardness might result in the total loss of an eye. He has taken a complete medical course, has been graduated with the degree of Doctor of Medicine, is licensed to practice as physician and surgeon in his state, and is competent to diagnose all known diseases of the eye.

By disease is meant any departure from the normal or healthy state. Some departures from health will be refractive only; that is, they will be related simply to the lens system of the eye. But other departures from health may be developmental, inflammatory, or a result of injury.

An ophthalmologist must also be able to tell when failing eyesight is due to poisons like methyl alcohol, to infections like syphilis, or to metabolic disease like nephritis (kidney disease). He must be able to use powerful drugs like atropine and cocaine, and must be adept at very delicate surgery like that required for the cataract operation.

By contrast with the above, the responsibilities of the optometrist are much more modest. He does not attempt to diagnose diseases like nephritis, nor to operate surgically for conditions like cataract, nor to treat infections like syphilitic iritis. An optometrist employs any means other than the use of drugs for the measurement of the powers of vision and the adaptation of lenses for the aid thereof.

The optometrist is trained to detect such conditions as nearsightedness and astigmatism, to determine their severity as far as is possible without the use of drugs, and to fit glasses in many cases when the only trouble is some peculiarity in the lens system of the patient's eye. By supplying well-fitting glasses he is commonly able to correct poor eyesight due to excessive or insufficient refraction (lens power) in an otherwise normal eye.

The third professional group to be mentioned here is that of the optician. An optician is one skilled in optics, that branch of physical science which treats of the nature and properties of light, the laws of its modification by opaque and transparent bodies, and the phenomena of vision. He is one who deals in optical glasses and instruments.

To merit the title of "optician" a student will generally complete a university course majoring in physics and will thereafter engage in teaching, research, or industrial work on optics. He may qualify for membership in professional societies, but there are no legal requirements, and he need not secure a state license in order to carry on his work.

It is evident that each of these three professional groups has special fields of activity, uses particular types of equipment, and has certain limitations.

The optometrist can help you to see better if there is no deep-lying disease or serious structural injury responsible for the impairment of vision. But if there is any reason to suppose that there is something seriously wrong, or that failing eyesight is related to disease in other parts of the body, clearly the training, experience, and equipment of the ophthalmologist render him best fitted to deal with the problem.

part 2: speech

16

speech disorders

Although speech disorders are often associated with serious loss of hearing, speech failure may also result from virus injury to the brain, as from German measles before birth. In this condition, known as controlled auditory imperception, the child may hear but is unable to interpret the meaning of sound and his speech suffers.

The child with a cleft lip and cleft palate has been injured during his embryological days before birth, with failure of tissues to fuse in a normal manner. The child with these gross anatomical defects is seriously handicapped in speech, psychological reactions, control of infections as well as normal development of the teeth and even in obtaining an adequate diet. Surgical corrections can be achieved in the early years.

Stuttering is primarily a functional disorder, although many speech disorders may have both organic or functional components. Causes of speech disorders are multiple and they may not always be apparent, even to the skilled diagnostician.

speech failure without deafness from german measles

Ames, Mary D., Stanley A. Plotkin, Richard A. Winchester and Thomas E. Atkins. "Central Auditory Imperception," Journal of the American Medical Association, 213: 419–421 (No. 3), July 20, 1970.

Two physicians and two research associates of the Children's Hospital in Philadelphia report that previous studies have shown that from 20 to 30 per cent of all infants are born deaf if their mothers have developed rubella (German measles) during pregnancy. It has been believed that this loss of hearing was due to destruction of the cochlea of the inner ear, so that sound could not be transmitted to the brain through the auditory nerve.

The four Philadelphia investigators report a study of 118 children who were not responding to sound, were not developing speech, or whose mothers had German measles during pregnancy. It was found that in 50 children the major cause of failure to learn to speak was deafness.

Thirty of the children, however, were found to have central auditory imperception with no associated damage of the mechanism that transmits sound to the brain. This is a condition in which there is an inability to respond appropriately to sound at the brain level. Such a child responds inconsistently to sound. At times he responds to the sound of the doorbell, the telephone, fire engines, airplanes and so on—but not always. He does not appear to listen and seems to ignore his native tongue because he does not understand it. The child fails to develop speech, and parents may think the failure is due to deafness.

Central auditory imperception is diagnosed by careful audiometric examination. Responses to pure tone by air and bone are normal or nearly normal. The blink which normally is obtained by a sudden loud noise at 80 decibels is not obtained except with greater intensity of sound. Painful hearing, which usually occurs at 120 decibels, is absent. The child shows little ability to localize sound. The electroencephalic (brain wave) response to sound is normal. Repeated tests are needed to confirm the diagnosis. In this study blood tests also revealed significant antibody levels for German measles (rubella). The child with central auditory imperception must be distinguished from the mentally retarded child and from the one who has had damage to peripheral hearing.

Early identification is important because treatment is different from that given other conditions. The child with speech impairment from mental retardation should be given training that helps him reach his maximum potential, limited though it may be. The child with damage to the inner ear or other parts of the system that conducts sound to the brain needs treatment by amplification of sound through use of hearing aids. In contrast, the child with inability to understand the meaning of sound must be educated to overcome his handicap. If this child's intelligence is in the normal range, he has the potential of good development if frustration and emotional reactions do not impair the potential before the nature of his problem is diagnosed properly.

A cooperative program involving the school district of Philadelphia and the Children's Hospital was started in 1970. The child is first taught to identify sounds in his environment, such as the telephone, the doorbell and so on in a quiet place. He is then taught to recognize the same sounds with background noise, such as music. He is then taught to localize the sound and to become aware of speech. Speech awareness is attained by getting the child's undivided attention in a quiet room and then talking to him directly in a loud tone or directly into his ear. Once speech awareness has been achieved, the child is then taught to produce speech by mimicking animals and the consonants of language. When the child is three or four years of age, the four investigators say, the elements of speech may be systematically introduced as McGinnis recommends. (McGinnis, M.A. *Aphasic Children Identification and Education by the Association Method,* Washington, D.C.: Alexander Graham Bell Association for the Deaf, 1963.) Teaching the child with congenital auditory imperception to speak is a very slow process.

speech disorders of children with cleft palate

Takagi, Yasuaki, Robert E. McGlone and Robert T. Millard. "A Survey of the Speech Disorders of Individuals with Clefts," Cleft Palate Journal, 2: 28-31, January 1965.

Two specialists from the National Institutes of Health and one from the Lancaster Cleft Palate Clinic of Lancaster, Pennsylvania report on a study of more than 1,000 persons with cleft lips and cleft palates over a period of 10 years.

Data acquired for the survey were obtained from speech evaluations written at the time of diagnosis. No distinction was made regarding the severity of the cleft lip or cleft palate.

Nearly 32 per cent of the afflicted persons were found to have adequate speech, despite their handicaps.

A combination of nasal tones and articulation defects occurred in nearly 28 per cent of the total group. Approximately 22 per cent more of the persons studied had nasal sounds alone. Another 17 per cent had defects of articulation alone. Thus, speech disorders involving nasality and articulation defects, alone or in combination, occurred in approximately 67 per cent of the 1,000 persons. Since approximately 32 per cent were found to have adequate speech, only 1 per cent of the group had other disorders of speech. Delayed speech was the leading handicap found in this remaining 1 per cent.

cleft lip and cleft palate

Crawford, Hugh H., Charles E. Horton, and Jerome E. Adamson. "Recent Advances in Cleft Lip and Cleft Palate Care," Virginia Medical Monthly, 93: 66–72, February 1966.

Three physicians of Norfolk, Virginia, with experience in plastic surgery, report that the problem of cleft lip and palate is very distressing. The parents and family are greatly disturbed by the appearance of this deformity, particularly in the more severe forms. It occurs in some form in approximately one in every seven hundred live births in all localities. Fortunately much can be done to correct deformities and give these children an opportunity for a normal life.

Although many questions remain unanswered as to the cause of this malformation, it is known that periods of stress and certain virus infections during the first three months of pregnancy are probable causes in some cases. Certain of the Vitamin B complex, including folic acid, provide some degree of protection against the occurrence of these deformities in a child born into a family in which a previous deformity has occurred. Heredity can be traced in approximately 20 per cent of the cases of cleft lip and palate.

In some instances, regardless of the diligent effort made to repair the palate, and even when blessed with excellent healing, the tissues available are insufficient to effect a sufficient closure for good speech. In such instances attempts to obtain better closure by surgery using other tissues is now being attempted with promising success. One such procedure is the transfer of throat tissues to the soft palate.

In general the cleft lip is repaired at about three to six weeks after birth, in two stages of surgery if necessary. This early repair of the cleft lip aids in molding the skeletal structures, improves the infant's ability to take feedings, and is a great psychological relief to the family. The positioning of the cleft segment is begun in infancy and closed with bone grafts at six to eight months of age, when the baby is capable of tolerating this somewhat more formidable procedure. The posterior palate cleft is repaired at about 18 to 24 months of age or before the beginning of speech.

Much can also be done for the older patient who had a cleft lip or palate or both repaired some 20 or 30 years ago, before the methods of repair were as refined as they are today. Some revision of the lip scar, a shift of tissue perhaps, or correction of an associated nose deformity can do much to decrease the disfigurement in such cases.

Possibly the most important recent development resulting in better overall care for these unfortunate individuals has been the use of a team approach in their care. Such a team consists of the reconstructive surgeon, an orthodontist, a speech therapist, a pediatrician, and a psychiatrist or social worker.

speech training of mothers

Sommers, Ronald K. "Factors in the Effectiveness of Mothers Trained to Aid in Speech Correction," Journal of Speech and Hearing Disorders, 27: 178-86 (No. 2), May 1962.

In Armstrong County, Pennsylvania half of eighty mothers of school children with articulation speech disorders of a functional nature received special training in the correction of speech defects. Mothers and children were both given speech, auditory discrimination and intelligence tests. The other 40 mothers were given no training.

The McDonald "Deep Test" of articulation was used for studying speech progress. Picture stimuli elicited spontaneous responses from the subjects for 11 consonant sounds. In this test a total of 631 misarticulations was possible for each person tested.

Speech results in children were compared between groups of mothers who received speech correction training and mothers who did not receive this training. The training of the mothers included 15 minutes per day in lectures, 15 minutes in discussions, 15 minutes in observations, and five minutes in demonstrations.

The program of training began with general introductory material that quickly evolved into specific problems to meet speech needs. Specific games and exercises were stressed for the mothers of children who were misarticulating the same words.

The children with articulation problems whose mothers received speech training showed significantly greater progress in the improvement of articulation. Children of normal intelligence showed greater improvement than slow learning children. Trained mothers showed nearly twice as much improvement in auditory discrimination as the untrained mothers and this improvement was definitely correlated with speech improvements of the child. This advantage prevailed regardless of whether group or individual training was given.

dangers of delayed speech therapy

Robert N. Plummer, "Dangers of Delaying Speech Therapy," Arizona Medicine, 13: 8–9 (No. 1), January 1956.

Robert N. Plummer, Ph.D., speech pathologist of Phoenix, Arizona, says that delay in seeking treatment for speech disorders may create serious problems. During a period of 15 years Dr. Plummer found that his patients averaged seven years of age, exclusive of adults. Dr. Plummer believes that an individual learns more speech from birth to age six than during any other six-year period. It is also easier for the defective child to achieve normal speech when he is given assistance during this speech development period.

A case in point concerns two brothers, one four and the other six years of age. The response of the younger child to speech therapy was amazingly faster than that of the older child. It can also be demonstrated that the early treatment of speech disorders enables a great majority of stutterers six years of age and under to be corrected within six months, while those over the age of six years require eight to ten months of treatment.

Another reason why the early treatment of disordered speech is important is the danger of psychological injury. Abnormal speech represents a glaring deviation from the normal. A speech disorder reaches its peak of seriousness when the child gets the idea that he is an abnormal individual.

If the child is fortunate enough not to recognize his defective speech as a handicap during the preschool period, he usually recognizes it as such upon entering school. Children strange to him are quick to point out his deficiency since they are brutally frank in pointing out abnormal deviations in others.

Parents seek delay in treatment because nearly everyone believes that his child will outgrow the speech failure. This attitude constitutes the greatest problem the speech defective faces in securing relief from his handicap. Not only does a trust exist among parents, but this is strengthened by advice from friends, neighbors, relatives, and other associates. While it is true that some children do outgrow defective speech, the assumption that all will do so is proven false every day.

Extensive testing by the writer in 20 Phoenix elementary schools and in the training school at Arizona State College at Tempe reveals that 22 per cent of all first graders in these schools had defective speech. It was also revealed that 18 per cent of all eighth graders were speech defective. This indicates a relatively small decline over this period of eight years.

The parents, the schools, and every agency which contacts the speech defective must be alerted to the urgency of early treatment of speech disorders.

cancer of the vocal cords

Shaw, H. J. "Glottic Cancer of the Larynx," Journal of Laryngology and Otology, 79: 1–14 (No. 1), January 1965.

A London physician reports on ten years of medical, surgical and radiological treatment of cancer of the vocal cords at the Royal National Throat, Nose and Ear Hospital. The report pertains to 306 patients with cancer of the vocal cords.

Hoarseness was present in all patients for one month to 10 years before hospital admission. Chronic inflammation of the larynx was apparantly responsible for hoarseness preceding the onset of cancer. Other leading symptoms were persistent cough, pain in the throat or ear, difficult breathing and discomfort in the throat.

In most cases the cancer was limited to a part of one vocal cord. Treatment by radiation or surgery resulted in five-year cures in about 62 per cent of all the patients, but about 85 per cent were cured if the vocal cord only was involved.

Cancer of the vocal cords appears to have a better chance of cure than other mucosal cancers of the head and neck.

speech-handicapped children

Duffy, Edward P., Jr. "Speech Handicapped Children," Journal of the Medical Society of New Jersey, 50: 26–31 (No. 1), January 1953.

Edward P. Duffy, Jr., M.D., of Belville, New Jersey, says that failure on the part of children to speak normally may be due to congenital deafness because of German measles of the mother during pregnancy, untreated syphilis, ear infections, meningitis, inflammation of the brain, tumors, and other diseases. Failure to speak may also be due to mongolism and mental retardation as well as other reasons.

Children in a nonstimulating speech environment may be of superior intellect and still not talk. When these children begin to acquire speech they do so rapidly. Sometimes parents, relatives, or brothers and sisters may anticipate the wants of a child to such an extent that there is no need for him to learn to speak.

Defects of the tongue, lips, jaw, or teeth (which affect chiefly the enunciation of consonants) cause disorders of articulation. Some children have these disorders because of neuromuscular disease. There is a widespread misconception that tongue-tie is a common source of speech defects. Regressive speech and infantile patterns of speech are due to other factors in the great majority of cases.

Disorders of phonation result from deformities and diseases of the nose, palate, uvula, and larynx, which interfere with the sounding of vowels. Disorders of pitch, tone, tempo, and intensity of speech are expressions of emotionally conditioned sounds. Tumors of the vocal cords may also cause phonation disorders. Conduction deafness, infection of the middle ear, nerve deafness, inflammation of the brain, head injuries, and a variety of other disorders may cause phonation defects.

Disorders of rhythm in speech, such as stuttering, are usually related to the environment of the person affected. There is no congenital deformity which has been proved to be the cause of stuttering.

Disorders of comprehension are based upon a lack of understanding language. Chronic diseases are often a factor in this type of speech disorder. Sometimes lack of comprehension may result from frequent school absences. Children with word deafness, even when they are of normal intelligence, will have great difficulty in adjusting to the world because they do not comprehend it. Adjustments without psychiatric help are difficult.

Sensory or receptive aphasia is a disturbance in which other people's languages are not comprehended. Motor or expressive aphasia does not reflect mental deficiency, and the outlook is good if the child has already acquired speech. Sometimes brain pathways may be injured by a brain abscess or some other condition so that the child can understand but cannot speak.

Psychotic children will not benefit from speech therapy alone. The child with schizophrenia has the speech tools, vocabulary, and even the grammar necessary for adequate speech but is apt to be completely unintelligible most of the time because he lives in a world of fantasy.

hygiene of the voice

Editorial. "Hygiene of the Voice," Journal of the American Medical Association, 135: 1154–55 (No. 17), December 27, 1947.

An editorial in the *Journal of the American Medical Association* points out that a defect of speech is a mental, social, and economic handicap, which often results in embarrassments and disturbances in family, industrial, and public life. Many scientists are convinced that the factors involved in speech difficulties are primarily mental or emotional.

Functional impediments to speech, such as chronic hoarseness and voice weakness, may be due to phobias resulting in over-or-under-activity of the vocal apparatus. Overuse produces the impression of strain; underuse an impression of flabbiness.

Froeschels found that 93 per cent of the preschool children in Vienna had hoarse voices. He examined the voices of 1,000 school children while they were speaking and while they were reading. The few who did not show straining of the voice during speaking showed it during reading. The slight emotion produced by the difficulties which reading offers a child seems to be one of the reasons for the sudden increase in hyperfunction.

Froeschels describes an original method of treating functional disturbances of voice which he designates as the chewing method. The idea is based on the observation that one can chew, speak, and even sing at the same time. Long observation convinced Froeschels that chewing was the origin of human speech.

Many people when chewing with the mouth open have the tongue continually on the floor of the mouth but that, according to Froeschels, is not the way savages chew: they lift and drop the tip of the tongue. Only the original method of chewing guarantees the setting free of the voice.

The patient is advised to chew with voice production at least twenty times a day for a few seconds only, but should always avoid doing so mechanically. He should act with the guiding idea of having some food in his mouth. After a few days he should read several times a day for one or two minutes only but should begin with a voiced "nonsense" chewing, and should always, after having read some words, introduce another "nonsense" chewing.

Dr. Chevalier Jackson notes that one of the pitfalls in the treatment of voice weakness is the belief that some different system of vocal training or some special exercises will cure the overworked muscles. He feels that absolute rest is necessary before any new system of training is undertaken so that the muscles may recover from the damage previously done. His plan includes a period of absolute silence at least half as long as the duration of the strenuous use of the voice; next, omission of any use of the voice on days when there is especially strenuous vocal work; he recommends absolute silence on the weekend and elimination of all attempts to talk against noise. Any necessary use of the telephone is to be done with a low voice and with the telephone transmitter held close to the lips. Especially dangerous is an attempt by singers or public speakers to extend the range of pitch upward.

More study is needed on both the hygiene of the voice and the technics desirable to strengthen and prolong its function.

causes of speech defects

Perkins, William H. and Richard F. Curlee. "Causality in Speech Pathology," Journal of Speech and Hearing Disorders, 34: 231-238 (No. 3), August 1969.

Two speech specialists of the University of Southern California in Los Angeles discuss a controversial issue when they consider the causes of speech disorders. Various theories have been advanced as major causes of speech defects or disorders of communication. In the professional literature the causes of speech disorders have been described as being due to: 1) some preceding experience, such as a brain injury to the left temporal lobe of the brain; 2) some characteristic of the individual; 3) mental retardation or some other phenomenon that causes delayed speech and language development; 4) some single aspect such as excessive muscle tension of the larynx that causes tense speech; or 5) a characteristic of the speech system, such as pitch being caused by the frequency of the vocal tone.

Methods of investigation of causes limit the conclusions that can be drawn. In speech defects, cause and effect can never be determined with absolute certainty. The possibility remains that an unobserved cause may remain. The best that science can provide is an explanation that is highly probable.

Any speech disorder is apt to be both organic and functional. Persons with cerebral palsy, aphasia (defect in or loss of the power of expression by speech) or cleft palate are still capable of wide ranges of speech responses despite their handicaps. To say their responses are limited by their handicaps is not necessarily to say that such handicaps cause their limitations.

It would be an awesome task for anyone to describe a single sound in relationship to neurological, respiratory, auditory, phonatory, articulatory, and other relationships. Over 100 muscles must receive messages from the brain (neural orders) whether to relax, contract, or maintain tonus at a rate suitable for the regulation of normal speech. The complexity of trying to describe speech on a physiological basis is staggering.

No level of abstraction can claim superiority as an explanation of a cause of speaking behavior.

If our knowledge of disorders of communication were extensive and exact and treatment so exact that we could modify defective speech with certainty, then specialists in speech could perhaps afford the luxury of loose logic, but muddled thinking about cause and effect in speech defects preserve conceptions for which speech specialists hold professional responsibility. Causes of speech disorders are not always apparent.

one thousand stutterers

Robbins, Samuel D. "1000 Stutterers: A Personal Report of Clinical Experience and Research with Recommendations for Therapy," Journal of Speech and Hearing Disorders, 29: 178–186 (No. 2), May 1964.

A speech specialist with a lifetime of clinical experience in working with stutterers has summarized the important points in treatment of this disorder.

If a young child begins to stutter, the parents should completely ignore the stuttering. They should show no annoyance, but should show the best example of calm, normal speech, in low-intensity, deliberate, and short sentences.

If the stutterer blocks on some word when asking a question, the parent should frame the answer so as to begin with the word by which the child stutters, being careful to prolong in a low-pitched voice, the first vowel in that word. No treatment should be attempted unless the young stutterer becomes sensitive to the fact that he stutters and begins to block on difficult words.

A child must learn never to fight his stuttering. Although he has learned to push harder if a door does not open, he must learn that in stuttering, pushing harder on muscles that are already tense or locked in spasm does no good. The child must learn to stop speaking the moment he feels a block approaching. Once he has stopped he must learn not to be in a hurry to resume speaking.

Dr. Robbins describes a "voice-sigh" technique that he has found to be effective in relaxing and retraining the stutterer in the use of his vocal cords. The details of this technique should be studied in full.

Studies show that stutterers are apt to be excessively sensitive to criticism. The child is apt to mirror the family. A tense child often reflects a tense family background; many have been violent family quarrels. Parents should be taught to ignore completely, for at least one year, any non-fluency in the speech of the child. The majority of stutterers are inclined to feel inferior and they lack self-confidence. Parents should speak softly to them, love them, and build up their confidence with praise for good work, whatever it is.

stuttering

Counihan, Donald. "Stuttering: Etiology and Prevention," Clinical Pediatrics, 3: 229–32 (No. 4), April 1964.

An Associate Professor of Communication Disorders at the University of Oklahoma Medical Center in Oklahoma City says that stuttering still continues to be poorly understood. Treatment plans have emphasized changing the child's habitual handedness, referring him for psychiatric treatment, following elaborate systems for developing "confidence," and many other procedures. Fortunately, a profound dissatisfaction with this state of affairs has led researchers to move in a different direction.

Most cases of stuttering are diagnosed between the second and fifth years of life, during the speech learning period. The first stages probably represent no more than normal failure to master the sensory-motor integrations required for speech. Breakdowns in fluency usually occur when the child is excited or under stress. At first the child is not aware of his non-fluency, but when he develops the awareness he learns to distrust his speech skills.

Recent research reveals that children who stutter do so on the same sounds, words, and phrases. Young stutterers soon learn to anticipate trouble.

When parents are convinced that the child's speech is normal, their anxiety often subsides, and the child is given opportunity to develop fluency without pressure. If the child shows consistent word fears and other symptoms of early stuttering, then his environment must be modified if improvement is to occur. Early treatment is directed against the child's environment rather than against the child. The aid of the parents must be enlisted in discovering the situations that precipitate stuttering. Parents are advised to allow the child ample time to speak, to avoid communicating to the child any embarrassment that they may feel, to maintain normal eye-contact with the child while he is speaking, and to avoid suggestions to the child that he modify his speech in any way. If the child feels that he is falling short of parental expectations he is apt to develop anxiety and further speech difficulty. Parents are urged to encourage the child to speak when tension is absent and when he appears to have greatest fluency. Speech is only one part of behavior and the child should not get the idea that it is the only aspect of his personality that deserves comment. Tension in other phases of the child's life must be minimized also. If stuttering is treated early it can usually be resolved.

causes of defective speech

Laguaite, Jeanette K. "Causes of Defective Speech in Children: Analysis of 140 Cases," Journal of the Louisiana State Medical Society, 107: 119–21 (No. 3), March 1955.

Jeanette K. Laguaite, Ph.D., assistant professor of speech pathology at Tulane Medical School in New Orleans, reports a study of the causes of defective speech in 140 cases.

The 140 children with speech defects were seen at the Speech and Hearing Center over a two-year period from March 1952 to March 1954.

The defective speech cases were divided into two broad groups: 1) those who were not able to communicate at all by means of speech or who could say only one or two words, and 2) those with some language development but whose speech was characterized by so many omissions, substitutions, and distortions of sounds as to be almost entirely unintelligible.

Approximately 47 per cent of the children were diagnosed as having functional speech disorders. This term was applied to those cases in which no disease or pathology could be demonstrated and in which the failure to speak seemed to be traceable to a simple failure to learn the correct patterns of normal speech.

In the order of frequency of occurrence, mental retardation accounted for 40 per cent of the speech defects, hearing loss accounted for 39 per cent of speech disorders, and emotional disturbances were involved in 20 per cent of the cases. These were the three leading causes responsible for the lack of development of speech in this study.

It was estimated that in less than one-half of the 81 cases of defective speech and in none of the 59 cases of no speech would the child be expected to overcome his handicap without some special treatment.

part 3: hearing

17

hearing losses and deafness

Deafness shuts out much of the world for the afflicted individual. He has difficulties in expression and problems in the acquisition of knowledge. His communication with others is seriously impaired. Socially and psychologically the one who is deaf stands apart from those around him. The beauty of music is not for him. Learning is more difficult, employment harder to secure and the pleasure of human relationships arduous to sustain. Perhaps most of those who are deaf cannot have hearing restored to them. Social and psychological rehabilitation may be their most fundamental needs.

life problems of deaf people

Switzer, Mary E. and Boyce R. Williams. "Life Problems of Deaf People," Archives of Environmental Health, 15: 249-256 (No. 2), August, 1967.

Two members of the Vocational Rehabilitation Administration in Washington, D.C. report that approximately one person in 700 is deaf in the United States. The hearing loss of deaf people is generally irreversible, whereas persons who are hard of hearing can almost always be helped medically. Deaf people stand apart from the general population psychologically and socially.

When hearing disappears the individual's environment shrinks enormously. He is not warned of dangers beyond his vision. The sound of beautiful music is not for him. The absorption of news and knowledge through lecture, radio, or conversation is impossible. He is in deep isolation in a milling crowd.

Many deaf people are without useful speech despite years of training. Most deaf people have normal strength, agility and intelligence, but serious communication difficulties create psychosocial problems. Deaf people are underinvolved in the mainstream of life, have limited sharing with their fellow men, have difficulties in being accepted by their families, neighbors, and employers.

The problem of communication has two aspects: 1) deficiencies in transmitting thoughts and 2) deficiencies in receiving them. A few deaf people speak, read, and write almost normally because they suffered deafness after having learned language and speech patterns. The large bulk of deaf people speak, read, and write quite poorly and few people can understand them.

Because of their normal strength and intelligence and background of considerable shop training in schools for the deaf many deaf people can find work readily. However, they are often employed at levels well below their capacities so that serious underemployment is a major life problem for most deaf people, and especially for the highly intelligent ones.

hearing defects

Shambaugh, George E., Jr., "Recognition and Management of Hearing Defects," Postgraduate Medicine, 33: 139–41 (No. 2), February 1963.

Moderate impairment of hearing in the child who hears well enough to learn speech is apt to be undetected by the child himself and by the parents, who often consider the child as disobedient or stupid when he fails to respond or responds incorrectly. To detect these moderate hearing losses, routine testing of all school children is essential for many of the hearing losses are remediable.

High pitched hearing losses in adults are seldom recognized until the hearing deficiency affects the conversational range. In noisy occupations regular testing of hearing is important to detect this type of loss.

Hearing tests can classify impairments into 3 groups of hearing losses:

(1) Disorders of the outer or middle ear that obstruct the conduction of sound to the auditory nerve.

(2) Injury to nerve tissue in the inner ear or the brain.

(3) Impairment of conduction of sound combined with deterioration of nerve tissue.

Nearly all losses in group 1 can be corrected.

Losses in group 2 may be caused by congenital factors, old age, occupational noise, virus diseases such as mumps and damage from treatment with antibiotics. The antibiotics that are most apt to cause deafness are neomycin, kanamycin, streptomycin and especially dihydro-streptomycin (which even in small dosage may cause injury after a delay of several weeks to four months). Losses in group 2 cannot be improved except in the case of Ménière's disease which is a type of hearing loss associated with attacks of vertigo. When seen early, Ménière's disease can usually be controlled by nicotinic acid, injections of dilute histamine, limitation of dietary salt and omission of smoking.

Losses in group 3 may sometimes respond partially to appropriate surgery.

Now about 90 per cent of otosclerotic (bone growth against the stapes) patients with pure conductive losses can be restored to near-normal or normal hearing by surgery. Most progressive hearing impairments of the conductive type are due to otosclerosis. The operating microscope has brought about great improvement in technique.

loss of hearing

Richard H. Wehr and Marshall A. Becker, "Loss of Hearing: the Patient and His Problem," Ohio State Medical Journal, 52: 709-13 (No. 7), July 1956.

Richard H. Wehr, M.D., and Marshall A. Becker, of the Ohio State University and the Columbus Hearing Society, respectively, say that to understand the problems of the person with impaired hearing, we are forced to generalize about some of the dynamics of human behavior.

In children who have had substantial hearing losses from early life, we may find any or all of the following characteristics: 1) irritability and frustration; 2) anxiety in social situations; 3) suspicion; and 4) negative self-concepts.

The family plays a primary part in the effect of hearing losses upon children. The most fundamental objective is not speech itself, although speech becomes an important means toward socialization and growth of personality, which is the primary objective that should be sought.

The loss of hearing gives rise to many problems. Otologists are not only treating the physical problem today, but are counseling with patients at a most crucial time in their lives. Audiologists are developing new testing techniques and are offering special training programs designed to make adjustment to hearing loss as easy as possible. Educators are increasing the scope of training programs for the hearing-handicapped child, and electronic engineers, psychologists, and researchers are all participating in the attack on hearing loss. With such a team approach, it seems reasonable to forecast a broadening and more intelligent understanding and acceptance of hearing loss.

deafness in children

Dwyer, Gregory K. "Serous Otitis Media and Deafness in Children," Connecticut State Medical Journal, 21: 102–3 (No. 2), February 1957.

Gregory K. Dwyer, M.D., of the Yale University School of Medicine, reports that insidious hearing loss in children, with or without ear pain, is becoming more prevalent today. An important factor in this hearing loss is serous otitis media.

Serous otitis media may be described as an exudate or transudate in the middle ear caused by obstruction of the eustachian tube by edema, infection, or lymphoid tissue. Some investigators believe that allergy plays a major factor in this condition. Other investigators have found only a sterile fluid, but no laboratory evidence to support allergy, bacterial or viral infection in this type of ear disorder.

The condition usually develops after repeated bouts of "otitis" with pain or fever or deafness in any combination. Usually an antibiotic has been given for the ear disorder, after which the symptoms subside, only to recur shortly after the stopping of medication. In older children the complaint may be simply a plugged feeling or "water in my ear" condition.

Treatment of the chronic or recurrent type of serous otitis media is primarily directed toward removal of the fluid. This report involves 33 patients ranging in age from six months to 11 years on whom myringotomy and aspiration of the exudate were done in every case. Usually this treatment was accompanied by the removal of adenoids and tonsils. In a short two-year follow-up, only three patients of the total group were found to have had any recurrence of ear pain or deafness. In these three children the symptoms were milder, less frequent, of shorter duration, and responded to simple treatment.

A problem in carrying out a necessary myringotomy is that of overcoming the fear and reluctance of parents that the child will have a permanent "perforated ear drum," or that the child will have his hearing further destroyed by the procedure. This, of course, is not the case, and the greater hazard is that there may be a permanent hearing loss in adulthood if such treatment is not utilized.

conduction deafness

MacCready, Paul B. "Conduction Deafness in Children," Connecticut State Medical Journal, 16: 252–56 (No. 4), April 1952.

Paul B. MacCready, M.D., of New Haven, Connecticut, reports a study of conduction deafness in four hundred children, ranging in age from three to twelve years.

There are three common types of damage in the ear that result in conduction deafness, according to Dr. MacCready. Fixation of the bones that transmit sound in the middle ear may result from adhesions following infections, from chronic infections of the middle ear, or from stoppage of the Eustachian tube leading to the middle ear from the throat. Any damage which causes obstruction of the Eustachian tubes will interfere with normal movements of the small bones which transmit sound. In conduction deafness of every type, hearing is better by bone than by air. This is the reverse of the normal situation.

In this study it was found that conduction deafness in children was much more common than is usually suspected. The disorder occurred in 25 per cent of the children who had been referred for special study and probable tonsil and adenoid surgery.

In approximately 80 per cent of the cases, conduction deafness cleared up following removal of the tonsils and adenoids. Radium treatment was also helpful in restoring hearing.

emotional aspects of hearing loss

Knapp, Peter Hobart. "Emotional Aspects of Hearing Loss," Psychoso-matic Medicine, 10: 203-22 (No. 4), July-August 1948.

Peter Hobart Knapp, M.D., of the Psychiatric Department of the Harvard Medical School, reports a study of 510 patients from an Army Hearing Rehabilitation Service in respect to the relationship of hearing loss to psychiatric disability.

Various psychological relationships to loss of hearing were revealed. About 5 per cent of the group reacted to their condition by denying any hearing loss, overcompensating, withdrawing from association with others, or experiencing various other forms of neurotic behavior. About 3 per cent of the group welcomed their hearing loss in part. Nearly 6 per cent of the total group developed a loss in hearing because of a psychogenic disorder. Following confirmation of the emotional nature of the hearing loss by use of the galvanic skin resistance and other tests, effective cures were obtained by psychiatric treatment, including the use of sodium pentothal.

It appeared from this study that there was no single "psychology of deafness" but that people react in various ways to defend themselves against a hearing loss. On the other hand, it is evident that in some cases deafness is psychological in origin and must be treated by the psychiatric approach.

beethoven's deafness

Stevens, Kenneth M. and William G. Hemenway. "Beethoven's Deafness," Journal of the American Medical Association, 213: 434-37 (No. 3), July 20, 1970.

Two physicians from the Division of Otolaryngology at the University of Colorado Medical Center in Denver observe that very few illnesses have created such interest and speculation as Beethoven's deafness. However, the exact nature of his deafness remains unidentified. His grave has been opened twice in an attempt to provide an answer.

Beethoven's deafness began at age 27 in his left ear when he contracted severe diarrhea which continued on and off for six years. Beethoven felt that his hearing difficulties resulted from this disease, which was assumed to be typhoid fever. He described high-tone hearing loss associated with severe buzzing and whistling, as well as an intolerance to loud sounds.

Beethoven used various devices to aid his hearing. He found ear trumpets of limited value, but used them extensively. Another device he used was a wooden "drumstick," one end of which he held between his teeth while resting the other end on his piano. When used, this rod would allow hearing via bone conduction.

The hearing loss progressed slowly but steadily until the age of 52 when for practical purposes Beethoven was totally deaf. His speech, however, remained intact.

The authors feel that Beethoven's deafness can be explained most logically by a diagnosis of cochlear otosclerosis (a formation of spongy bone in certain parts of the ear, resulting in progressive deafness). This diagnosis fits with Beethoven's specific type of hearing loss and the majority of findings in the autopsy. Had Beethoven lived today, his hearing probably could have been improved through surgery.

When Beethoven's grave was opened and the skull examined, it was found to be in nine pieces with the temporal portions conspicuously absent. They had evidently been removed for study at an earlier time, and have never been located.

deafness in the infant

Illingworth, R. S. "The Child at Risk of Deafness," Clinical Pediatrics, 3: 510–11 (No. 9), September 1964.

A physician of the University of Sheffield in England says that it is particularly important to diagnose a hearing defect early, in order that the residual hearing can be utilized properly to enable speech to develop. Absence of speech makes early communication by the child impossible; he feels thwarted and isolated, and may well develop troublesome behavior problems.

It has been shown that any of the conditions listed below will reveal more than 14 times the incidence of deafness in the population as a whole. The relevant conditions follow:

Family history of deafness
Certain rare congenital disorders
Rubella (German measles) in first 3 months of pregnancy
Cretinism (a disease due to thyroid deficiency)
Cleft palate
Prematurity
Anoxia (lack of oxygen) at birth
Hyperbilirubinemia (an excess of certain bile pigments in the blood) in newborn period

Cerebral palsy
Mental subnormality
Ototoxic (poisonous or injurious to hearing) drugs—neomycin, vancomycin, kanamycin, viomycin, intrathecal dihydro-streptomycin
Purulent (pus producing) or recurrent otitis media (middle ear infection)

By far the most important of these clues is suspicion of deafness by the parents, and delayed or indistinct speech. A family history of congenital deafness is obviously important, but this is rare. Every child with indistinct speech, or speech which is retarded in relation to other aspects of the child's development, should have his hearing tested by an audiometrician. When rubella (German measles) occurs in the first three months of pregnancy, the risk of deafness is considerable. In a series of 57 children, there was a hearing defect in 30 per cent.

Testing of hearing in the first three months of life is not easy. For parents or non-medical personnel it depends on the following responses to a loud sound.

(1) A quieting of activity

(2) A catch in the respiration

(3) Blinking of the eyelids

(4) Crying (sometimes)

After the age of three or four months, the important response is the turning of the head towards a sound. Suitable stimuli which cover high tones and which are readily available are:

(1) Crumpling of tissue paper

(2) A high-pitched rattle

(3) A plastic spoon in a cup

(4) A toy hand bell

The sound stimulus must be applied out of the child's sight, close to the ear and on a level with it.

It must be remembered that a mentally subnormal child is late in all aspects of development, except occasionally gross motor development. It follows that he will be late in turning his head to sound. For instance, whereas the age at which a normal child begins to turn his head to sound averages three months, a child with a developmental quotient of 50 is not likely to turn his head to sound until he is six months old.

kidney diseases and loss of hearing

Nichol, K. P., and A. Miller. "Hereditary Nephritis and Deafness," The Journal-Lancet. 85: 236-240 (No. 6), June 1965.

Two members of the Department of Pediatrics of Marquette University School of Medicine in Milwaukee report that in recent years a disease that runs in certain families has been identified in which blood appears in the urine at intervals and there is a loss of hearing and defects of vision.

The authors studied 15 members of a particular family and found five of them with blood in the urine and other evidence of kidney disorder. Hearing tests were performed on 13 of the family members and hearing losses were detected, especially in the higher frequencies. At the time of the testing one male member of the family had blood in the urine and a hearing loss of 35 decibels at 1,000 cycles and a loss of 90 decibels at 6,000 cycles. A brother, who had no blood in his urine, had a hearing loss of 35 decibels at 1,000 cycles and a loss of 110 decibels at 4,000 cycles. Only one of the females in the family had a hearing loss which was compatible with her advancing age.

The cause of kidney damage was not established. In previous autopsy studies, connective tissue infiltration of kidney tissues appeared to be the most prominent finding.

The disease appears to be transmitted as a sex-linked dominant in which affected males cannot pass on the disorder to their sons, but could to all their daughters. An affected female can transmit the disease to either sons or daughters, half of them being affected by statistical expectancy.

otosclerosis

Francois, J., M. T. Matton–Van Leuven and P. Kluyskens. "Cytogenetic Study of Otosclerosis," Acta Geneticae Medicae et Gemellologiac. 16: 124-153 (No. 2), 1967.

Three Belgian scientists report a study in which 62 patients with otosclerosis were evaluated in terms of chromosome structures.

Otosclerosis is a disease of bone in which damage is limited to the bony capsule of the ear and to the middle ear bones. The most common localization of damaged bone is found in the area between the footplate of the stapes and the oval window.

The first signs of otosclerosis begin around the age of 20. The beginning destruction of the normal bone is characterized by a ringing in the ears (tinnitus) and is followed by progressive hearing loss.

It is thought that as long as the disease is limited to the oval window the deafness is classified as the conductive type. However, in 30 to 40 per cent of the cases the disease spreads into the cochlea (the essential and spiral part of the ear) and is then classified as perceptive or nerve deafness. In 59 of the 62 patients in this study the disease was present in both ears.

In this study the chromosomes were found to be normal and the scientists concurred with other investigators who have maintained that otosclerosis belongs to the group of genetic diseases characterized by mendelian inheritance rather than to any group caused by abnormal chromosomes.

inner-ear deafness of sudden onset

Lindsay, John R., and Jacob J. Zuidema. "Inner Ear Deafness of Sudden Onset," Laryngoscope, 60: 238–63 (No. 3), March 1950.

John R. Lindsay, M.D., and Jacob J. Zuidema, of Chicago, report sixteen cases of inner-ear deafness in which there was a sudden onset. In four cases the ear complication appeared to be associated with a general disease.

In one case the loss of hearing appeared to be due to a middle-ear infection. In another instance the loss of hearing appeared to be due to syphilis, and in still another case an inflammatory reaction of the auditory nerve appeared to be involved. The definite cause could not be ascertained in twelve cases. In three cases loss of hearing appeared to be associated with an inflammatory process of vision. In two of these there was a profound loss of hearing and disturbed function of balance.

sudden loss of hearing on one side

Jaffe, Burton F., Hunein F. Maassab. "Sudden Deafness Associated with Adenovirus Infection," New England Journal of Medicine, 276: 1406–1409 (No. 25), June 22, 1967.

A former physician resident of the University of Michigan Medical School and a member of the faculty of the University of Michigan School of Public Health report that the sudden loss of hearing on one side may be caused by a wide variety of medical and surgical diseases, such as blood clots, meningitis, syphilis, measles, mumps, multiple sclerosis, drugs, and other disorders.

This report gives documentary evidence of the first patient who suffered sudden deafness because of an Adenovirus infection. The offending virus was identified as Adenovirus Type 3. No case of sudden loss of hearing from this particular organism has been previously reported in the medical literature.

In this case a 38-year-old woman who developed a mild sore throat, nasal inflammation, and a slight cough had apparently caught a cold from her 4-year-old son who had been suffering from an acute upper respiratory tract infection. The mother first noticed a feeling of pressure and fullness in the left ear. Two hours later the hearing loss was severe and ringing in the ears was bothersome. She felt dizzy and had a feeling of congestion in the right ear without loss of hearing. At the time of medical examination she could still hear a whisper in this right ear, but could not hear a loud shout in her left ear.

Ordinarily, when there is a hearing loss associated with a cold, it is the middle ear that becomes congested and inflamed, so that sound is not conducted across this part of the hearing mechanism. However, in this patient, the loss of hearing was due to the virus infection in the inner ear where the acoustic nerve ends were invaded. The eardrum (tympanic membrane) was normal and there was no evidence that the middle ear was involved.

Sudden deafness should always be considered an emergency, because successful treatment and preservation of hearing depends on prompt therapy. One investigator has found that if the hearing loss is treated within four days that 62 per cent of the patients will recover; 47 per cent will recover if treatment is obtained within six weeks, but that practically no patient will recover his hearing if treatment is delayed longer than six weeks from the sudden loss of hearing. Under prompt and proper treatment recovery is usually complete within three or four weeks. In the patient reported here the good recovery had continued for nine months to the time of publication of this article, but the hearing level was not as good as in the uninvolved ear. Thus, there was some loss of hearing.

18

infections and hearing

Middle ear infection, once ranked as a cause of 50 per cent of all deafness in adult life, is still a major problem in childhood despite the antibiotics which are now highly effective against some invading organisms. Earache is still an emergency for which proper medical care should be secured and the neglected middle ear infection still carries the same hazard of the past so far as hearing is concerned. The accumulation of fluid in the middle ear, even though it is not infectious, may cause significant hearing loss. Infections of the throat are often involved in invasion of ear tissues and loss of hearing.

Cholesteatoma has been described as one of the most dangerous diseases involving the ear and one which may be associated with abscess formation and meningitis.

acute middle ear infections

Feingold, Murray, Jerome O. Klein, Gilbert E. Haslam, Jr., Jeremiah G. Tilles, Maxwell Finland and Sydney S. Gellis. "Acute Otitis Media in Children," American Journal of Diseases of Children, 111: 361–365 (No. 4), April, 1966.

Six physicians of the Harvard Medical School report that acute infection of the middle ear presents one of the most frequent and perplexing infectious disease problems of childhood.

The present study was conducted on 90 children who had swollen ear drums and other evidence of middle ear infection. Since it is often difficult to identify the specific organism with which the child may be infected, because nose and throat cultures are often uninformative, the physicians in this study made a needle aspiration of the middle ear fluid in order to identify the germs involved.

Disease-producing bacteria were identified from these needle aspirations in 48 of the children. Diplococcus pneumonia was the most frequent organism found and Haemophilus influenzae was the next most frequent germ that was found.

Nose and throat cultures on the same children predominantly failed to identify the same bacteria as a cause of the middle ear infection.

Oddly enough, the body temperature of children with middle ear infections in whom no bacteria could be identified by taking fluid directly by needle aspiration through the ear drum was found to be higher on the average than in those cases where the bacteria could be identified. In the so-called "sterile" ear fluids the temperatures averaged 103 degrees F., which was higher than in the other children. Viruses, of course, may have been involved in these infections, without identification in the study.

Obviously, treatment of the child with a middle ear infection would be most effective if the physician is aware of the specific germ that is involved and can use an antibiotic or other substance that is known to be effective against this organism.

earache

Smith, E. John. "Earache," Canadian Medical Association Journal, 66: 234–37 (No. 3), March 1952.

E. John Smith, M.D., of Montreal, Canada, says that there are two important points to remember in regard to an earache: first, the severity of the earache may not be an indication of the severity of the disease that may be involved; and second, earache may be an early symptom of serious disease of the upper respiratory or digestive passages.

Earache may be caused by objects in the external ear. Beans, peas, and other such materials may absorb moisture, swell, and cause severe pain when lodged in the external ear. Other objects such as beads and stones may cause pain from mechanical irritation. Hard wax in the ear may also cause pain.

Infections of various parts of the ear are common. Pain may be intense in the case of a furuncle. This type of pain is accentuated by movements of the jaw. Hearing acuity may be unaffected.

Acute infection of the middle ear is probably the most common cause of earache. It is almost always secondary to a nose and throat infection. It usually occurs in children. In these days treatment with antibiotics or sulfa drugs is highly successful, although in some cases the disease may be resistant.

A reflex earache may occur because of the anatomical arrangement of the nerve supply to the ear. Any structure supplied by the fifth, seventh, ninth or tenth cranial nerves or by the second or third cervical nerves may be a source of referred pain to the ear. Thus pain may actually originate elsewhere, as in the parotid gland, nose, throat, tongue, teeth, larynx, or neck, but be felt in the ear because of reflex action.

infections of the middle ear

Philip Rosenblum, "Medical Aspects of Otitis Media," Illinois Medical Journal, 110: 12-13 (No. 1), July 1956.

Philip Rosenblum, M.D., senior attending pediatrician of the Michael Reese Hospital in Chicago, says that otitis media is still one of the most frequently encountered pediatric diseases.

Some pediatricians feel that this disease of the middle ear can always be treated medically, while many otologists consider it a surgical disease.

Many of the complications of otitis media such as meningitis, thrombosis of the dural sinuses, and abscess of the brain are seen rarely now, but they have not been eliminated entirely.

The most important predisposing factors in the cause of otitis media are bacterial and viral respiratory infections, allergies, sinusitis, and enlarged tonsils and adenoids. Infants and young children are more prone to this infection of the middle ear because the Eustachian tubes are more horizontal and practically as large as in older children. In some families enlarged tonsils and adenoids are present from birth.

It is important to educate the public that earache is a serious complaint and that medical advice should be sought early. When a child with otitis media is treated early by the physician with sulfa drugs or antibiotics most infections will subside without any trouble or complications. Surgery is indicated when the patient has a bulging eardrum. Many eardrums never return completely to normal when this surgery is not done. Many patients with otitis media who were treated only with medicines may retain serum in the middle ear and the drums may be distended for weeks. Some of these patients appear to encounter impaired hearing at a later date.

middle ear infections

Halsted, Crystie, Martha L. Lepow, Neron Balassanian, Joseph Emmerich and Emanuel Wolinsky, "Otitis Media," American Journal of Diseases of Children, 115: 542–551 (No. 5), May 1968.

Five physicians report from their experience and clinical research that middle ear infection (otitis media) is a common problem in infants and children.

Even though several antibiotics are effective in controlling the complications associated with the production of pus, middle ear infection is still a significant cause of illness and hearing loss.

Bacteriologic studies have shown repeatedly that in only 60 to 70 per cent of middle ear infections is it possible to identify the cause of the infection. Possibly viruses are responsible for the 30 to 40 per cent of cases where the germ cannot be identified. Few systematic attempts to isolate virus from middle ear fluid have been reported in the medical literature.

In this study 106 children from the age of two months to 5½ years with middle ear infections were studied. Most of these children had a bulging eardrum; in a few the eardrum was only diffusely red. In 65 of the children (61 per cent) the inflammation of the eardrums was on both sides, indicating that the middle ear infection involved both ears. 60 per cent of the children had previously experienced one or more episodes of middle ear infection.

Discharge from the nose and irritability of the child were the most common complaints at first. Specific symptoms relating to the ear were less common.

The results in this study confirm those of previous medical investigators, although the identification of the specific organism involved in the middle ear infection in only 60 per cent of the cases is slightly lower than some other physicians have reported. However, one-half of the patients with bacterial invasion of the middle ear also had evidence of virus or mycoplasma infections. Infections with these organisms may predispose to bacterial invasion of the middle ear.

Approximately 75 per cent of the young patients in this study showed rapid control of inflammation regardless of treatment. However, some would have benefitted by antibiotic treatment, and several children who received antibiotics did not recover promptly. There was a high recurrence of middle ear infection in some children even after successful treatment and it has been well documented that there is an increasing probability of hearing loss with repeated episodes of middle ear infections (otitis media).

Prevention appears to lie in the prevention of upper respiratory infections, which may become possible in the future with vaccines. The pneumococcus organism was found in the fluid drawn from the middle ear in 39 patients. In 19 more an influenza organism (H influenzae) was identified. These findings support the concept that some middle ear infections are preceded by upper respiratory infections.

hearing loss in school children

Herzon, E. M. "Respiration in School Children Recoverable Hearing and Nasal," Illinois Medical Journal, 111: 70–75 (No. 2), February 1957.

E. M. Herzon, M.D., of Elgin, Illinois, reports an analysis of 350 cases of hearing losses in school children. All of the hearing losses had been discovered by use of the audiometer.

It was found in this study that nine out of ten of the hearing losses were reversible, at least to the point where there was no residual, practical, hearing handicap. Of the 350 cases, 70 per cent were returned to normal hearing, and an additional 20 per cent were returned to normal hearing within the range of speech although some abnormalities were found in the higher tones.

After the use of planned ephedrine nose drops, 75 children returned to normal hearing within one to four weeks. Many of the remaining children needed surgical removal of adenoids and tonsils and in a few radium treatment was required. Of the entire group of children, only 8 per cent were left after treatment with a practical hearing loss. Of the 29 children who comprised this 8 per cent, there were 17 in whom the hearing returned to normal in one ear. This left only 12 children, or approximately 3.5 per cent of the total, with subnormal hearing within the speech range. Many of these children were found to be suitable prospects for hearing aids.

A functional nasal respiratory test was used as the diagnostic index in deciding whether medical or surgical treatment was needed for these hearing losses in children. Investigation showed that the lymphatics of the middle ear and eustachian tube played an important role in the hearing loss. There appeared to be an acquired respiratory nasal tissue sensitivity, or allergy, in many of the children.

fluids in the middle ear

Fitz-Hugh, G. Slaughter and Robert T. Stone. "Serous Otitis Media in Children," Virginia Medical Monthly, 93: 61–65 (No. 2), February 1966.

Two physicians of the Department of Otolaryngology of the University of Virginia Hospital in Charlottesville observe that non-pus-containing fluids in the middle ear have become relatively commonly diagnosed by doctors in the past 25 years. This condition, called serous otitis media by the two ear specialists, has many different names and the true causes of it are controversial. No single cause has been found in every case.

Malformations of the eustachian tube (the tube linking the middle ear and the throat) that cause poor ventilation and drainage of the middle ear cavity are almost always responsible for the condition. Many different factors can cause blocking of the eustachian tube, such as respiratory infections with enlarged adenoids, nasal allergy, dental malocclusion, malignancies of the nose or throat, cleft palate and other factors.

A mild to moderate hearing loss is associated with fluid in the middle ear, amounting only to about 10 to 15 decibels, but the loss is enough to retard academic and social development, the physicians believe.

Some authorities believe that antibiotics play a major role in the production of serous otitis media. Antibiotics are often given in the treatment of acute ear infections for too short a length of time and in inadequate doses. A smoldering infection may remain with production of a thick fluid somewhat like mucus.

The disease appears mostly in children between the ages of two and 15. The affected child has usually had several acute upper respiratory infections, mild earaches and treatment with antibiotics. Generally there is some hearing loss, but occasionally none at all. The child is usually restless, irritable, inattentive and deficient in school work. Often the classroom teacher is the first person to suspect the child has a hearing loss. Some children report a ringing in the ears. In small children the disease is often manifested by pulling on the affected ear, burying the head in a pillow on the affected side, or crying for no apparent reason. The audiogram usually shows a conductive hearing loss of 10 to 40 decibels.

Treatment calls for draining of the fluid from the middle ear and correction of the original cause, such as removal of the adenoids if they are involved. Sometimes the condition is allergic in origin and benefits may be derived from desensitization methods. If not corrected, the condition can lead to permanent hearing loss and disease of the mucous membranes of the middle ear.

cholesteatoma of the ear

Thomas, Gary L. "Cholesteatoma of the Ear," California Medicine. 108: 205–208 (No. 3), March 1968.

A physician of Sacramento, California says that cholesteatoma is one of the most dangerous diseases involved in the ear. Although the disease is not an infection in itself it causes a chronic infection of the middle ear and loss of hearing along with other serious complications. Cholesteatoma is a cavity in the middle ear space or the mastoid in which there is a lining of epithelium. This abnormal kind of tissue in the middle ear peels off and creates debris which often contains crystals of cholesterol. This material accumulates in the ear and promotes bacterial growth so that infections usually develop.

Destruction of tissue is slow and insidious and may proceed for many years. Drainage may take abnormal channels such as into the brain where an abscess, meningitis, paralysis and deafness may occur. Facial paralysis may be the first sign to cause real alarm. Pressure on the facial nerve causes inflammation, swelling, loss of blood supply and nerve damage that results in loss of function.

Middle ear drainage may be intermittent or persistent and the loss of hearing progresses to a minimum of a 60 decibel hearing loss. Complete destruction of hearing may occur. Sometimes pain is a complaint and dizziness occurs sometimes.

In most cases surgical correction of the condition is needed to preserve hearing and stop the disease.

dizziness and "ear stroke"

Lewis, Miles L. "The Problem of the Dizzy Patient," Journal of the Kentucky Medical Association. 63: 424–25 (No. 6), June 1965.

An assistant professor of otolaryngology at Tulane University School of Medicine observes that dizziness is one of the more common symptoms that brings a patient to his physician.

The most important system for maintaining equilibrium is the vestibular system. The most severe types of vertigo are produced by a disturbance of this system of the ear. Various conditions involving the ear and associated with dizziness are discussed by Dr. Lewis, but he says that the vast majority of persons with true vertigo have some interference with the blood supply to the labyrinth of the inner ear. An "ear stroke" is a very dramatic affair and is due to an abrupt deprivation of blood because of a blood clot or hemorrhage. The patient is seized with sudden vertigo (dizziness), nausea and vomiting, and if the cochlea is involved there will be profound tinnitus (ringing in the ear) and extreme loss of hearing in the affected ear. Any movement of the head produces more severe symptoms. Symptoms are apt to subside slowly over a period of two to four weeks, but mild dizziness on change of body position may persist for several months.

19

noise and hearing

Modern research has shown quite clearly that noise can cause serious impairment of hearing. The effects of rock–and–roll music have been found to be detrimental to hearing and to cause permanent damage to some persons. Loss of hearing because of gunfire has also been demonstrated. In industry the effects of working in a noisy environment have long been known and many states have established limits on the noise that workers can be legally exposed to within a specified number of hours. The need for education, especially of young persons, should be obvious if we are to prevent impairment of hearing in large segments of our society.

damage to hearing from rock-and-roll music

Dey, Frederick L. "Auditory Fatigue and Predicted Permanent Hearing Defects from Rock-and-Roll Music," New England Journal of Medicine, 282: 467–70 (No. 9), February 26, 1970.

A physician of New London, Connecticut agrees with those experts who believe that modern civilization produces noise that is damaging to hearing. Noise has been described as a different kind of "air pollution" that is especially applicable to rock–and–roll music. Only recently have researchers shown that certain music groups who use powerful electronic amplification damage not only their own hearing, but those of listeners as well.

People differ widely in their susceptibility to injury from noise. When loss of hearing does occur because of noise, it is apt to develop without early detection. Most persons who have normal hearing can suffer a permanent loss of about 25 decibels before it is detectable by standard speech audiometric examinations, according to Dr. Dey. The hearing loss may develop insidiously over a period of months. Enough cases of hearing loss appear to be related to rock–and–roll music to justify scientific studies of the matter.

Although rock–band musicians have reported ringing in the ears or a "sensation of fullness" lasting for eight hours to several days after being exposed to sound pressure levels of 110 to 120 decibels in the rehearsal room, it must be remembered that only the octaves from 300 to 4800 cycles per second are potentially dangerous to the ear. If a drumbeat reaches a level of 120 decibels it has no relevance to noise injury to the ear if the dominant frequencies are all less than 300 cycles per second.

In this study Dr. Dey investigates whether or not damage to hearing is truly produced by typical rock music, and if so, what percentage of young normal ears can be expected to suffer auditory fatigue and permanent injury to hearing. Tape recordings with a sound-level meter were made of rock music in a discotheque. Twenty-minute samples of the music were then played through a set of octave-band filters to determine the cycles per second at different decibel readings. Fifteen men aged 18 to 25 years were exposed to the music in one ear at different combinations of sound-pressure levels and duration of time, from 5 to 30 minutes. Hearing tests were carefully done before and after the rock music at levels from 1000 to 8000 cycles per second. Results were adjusted by logarithmic means to a two-hour period of exposure.

Dr. Dey concluded from his research that two persons in 100 would recover hearing far too slowly after listening for two hours to rock music at 100 decibels, but at 110 decibels about 16 per cent of the listeners would probably have permanent damage to hearing. The rock music heard in a typical discotheque is apt to be at a sound-pressure level of 110 decibels recorded at a distance of 30 feet from the loud speakers.

effects of rock-and-roll music

Lebo, Charles P., Kenward S. Oliphant and John Garrett. "Acoustic Trauma from Rock-and-Roll Music," California Medicine, 107: 378-380 (No. 5), November 1967.

Three members of a research team of the University of California School of Medicine observe that existing research suggests that deafness or loss of hearing in old age may be due in part to the accumulated effects of environmental noise.

In this investigation the three research personnel measured sound levels in two San Francisco Bay Area rock-and-roll establishments frequented almost exclusively by teenagers and young adults, many of whom fall into a group often designated as "hippies." In the musical presentations the main instruments used were amplified guitars and the percussion group.

Sound recordings were made of the noise generated at multiple locations throughout the hall in which the music was being produced. These recordings were later analyzed in a laboratory with technical equipment.

The sound measurements were compared with the standards established by Noise Control Safety Orders of the Department of Industrial Relations of the State of California. The state standards are based upon the amount of sound that can produce damage to hearing after certain periods of exposure.

Noise greater than 92 decibels in sound pressure composed of certain frequencies and sustained for a period of one hour will produce as much as a 40-decibel loss in approximately 10 per cent of the ears exposed, between five and 30 decibel loss in about 80 per cent of ears and will produce no change in about 10 per cent of the listeners.

In each of the rock-and-roll recordings the noise level reached the point of damage to the human ear, according to experience with industrial noise.

The investigators conclude that the noise levels produced by some rock-and-roll bands (which ranged from 105 to 122 decibels in contrast to the acceptable limit of 92 decibels in industry) unmistakably exceed levels considered safe for prolonged exposure.

The authors also conclude that the reduction of noise levels to safe levels for hearing would still permit enjoyment of the music.

loss of hearing from gunfire

Keim, Robert J. "Impulse Noise and Neurosensory Hearing Loss," California Medicine, 113: 16–19 (No. 3), September 1970.

A physician associated with the Los Angeles County-University of Southern California Medical Center observes that not many people know that being close beside or behind a gun when it is discharged may cause permanent loss of hearing.

Doctor Keim, an ear, nose and throat specialist, says the average sound level in the average city has increased a thousand fold in the past 30 years.

There are two types of noise, the steady-state and the impulse. The difference in duration of the noise is the key distinction. Most of the research has been done on steady-state noise and standards have been evolved. If a person is exposed to noise at levels of 85 decibels or more during an eight-hour period he is encountering a hazardous noise level. Ear plugs or ear muffs need to be worn if a person is exposed to 95 decibels or more over a working day.

Noise	Decibels
Breathing	10
Whispering	20
Low street noise	40-50
Conversation	60-70
Food blender	88
Jack-hammer	94
Power mower	107
Motorcycle	110
Discotheque	110-120
Jet airplane at takeoff	150
Small firearms	140-160

Gunfire represents the impulse type of noise in which swift and acute exposure to noise occurs.

Some protection against noise of the steady–state type can be achieved by contraction of middle ear muscles that dampen the mobility of the tympanic membrane (eardrum) and the attached ossicles (small bones), but the amount of time needed is about 100 to 150 milliseconds. In gunfire noise reaches a peak intensity within about 2 milliseconds so there is not sufficient time for the body to protect itself.

Dr. Keim reports a study of 14 men who were exposed to gunfire and had a feeling of fullness, ringing in the ears and subjective hearing loss. All of the men were given hearing tests and found to have suffered damage of a permanent type to the auditory nerve. Most of the damage was above the

2,000 cycle level so that a long time might elapse before communication might be affected (most conversations occur between 500 and 2,000 cycles per second) so the hearing loss would be recognized.

hearing losses in high school musicians and riflemen

Corliss, Leland M., Mildred E. Doster, Jane Simonton and Marion Downs. "High Frequency and Regular Audiometry among Selected Groups of High School Students," Journal of School Health, 40: 400-405 (No. 8), October 1970.

Two physicians and their research associates of the Health Services of the Denver, Colorado Public Schools and the University of Colorado Medical School report a study of 1,000 high school students in respect to noise exposures and loss of hearing.

A questionnaire was used to explore ear health and exposure to noise. Then hearing levels were tested in two ways by means of the use of a regular audiometer and by use of a machine that measures high sound ranges (the Tracor Rudmose H.F. Machine, produced by the Tracor Company of Austin, Texas) of 4,000 to 18,000 Hz (high frequencies).

Fourteen of the 24 musicians who played in electric bands and 11 members of a rifle team passed the regular hearing tests of the standard audiometer, although 75 per cent of the musicians and 63 per cent of the riflemen had hearing losses that were revealed only by testing with the Tracor machine. Larger groups of musicians and riflemen were then tested. It was found that musicians began to deviate in their hearing at levels of 10,000 Hz, whereas riflemen began to show differences at 12,000 Hz.

The investigators concluded that hearing losses are very serious and probably permanent when young people are exposed to noise above 10,000 Hz. Ten boys with severe hearing loss were all involved in shooting, either on the rifle team or in hunting.

Fifty per cent or more of the hearing losses would not have been detected if testing had been restricted to use of the regular audiometer only.

The investigators recommend that schools should test hearing in the higher sound ranges up to 18,000 cps (cycles per second) and that educational measures should be promoted on hazards to hearing and the value of ear protectors and that there should be improved supervision of young people in respect to noise exposures.

cultural factors in hearing loss

Rosen, Samuel, Dietrich Plester, Aly El-Mofty, and Helen V. Rosen. "Relation of Hearing Loss to Cardiovascular Disease," Transactions, American Academy of Ophthalmology and Otolaryngology, 68: 433–44 (No. 3), May–June 1964.

Three physicians from New York City, Dusseldorf, and Cairo collaborated in studies with others to assess more accurately the effect of aging on hearing. Research started in 1961 to study the hearing of a population living in a noise-free environment (it is known that constant noise has an adverse effect on hearing, which would make it difficult to differentiate the effects of aging). Such a population, the Mabaans, was found living in a remote region of Africa, 10 degrees above the equator.

The Mabaans were given hearing tests, heart examinations, blood pressure tests, blood cholesterol studies, and electrocardiographic examinations. The findings on the Mabaan tribe were compared with those of apparently healthy adults in the United States, whose life histories showed a minimum exposure to noise.

The hearing of the Mabaans was found to be markedly superior to that of the Americans. In Americans, there is a sharply increasing loss of hearing with each decade of life, particularly at the high frequencies. In contrast, all the Mabaan decade groups from the 10-year-olds through the 79-year-olds fell within the first two decade groups of the American group studied.

That noise may be a factor in explaining the poorer hearing in our culture seems fairly clear. But other factors probably play a much more significant role, such as vascular changes, diet, nutrition, stress and strain, metabolic imbalance, climate, and genetic factors.

It was found that high blood pressure and coronary heart disease are virtually unknown among the Mabaans, and there is very little hardening of the arteries. There is almost no fat in the Mabaan diet, and they are lean at all ages.

As part of this study, a comparison was made with the hearing of the East Finnish population (which has notoriously high blood cholesterol levels and one of the highest incidences of atherosclerosis and coronary heart disease in the world).

The diminishing hearing of the Finns in the age range from 14 to 29 years may already reflect the beginning of a long vascular process leading to atherosclerosis and coronary heart disease. It may be possible, therefore, for a high frequency hearing test to reveal such a trend in a population many years before the irreversible clinical vascular picture becomes manifest. Time and more studies of this kind are needed.

The role of circulatory factors in hearing loss may be considered to be related to the following factors:

(1) Diminished blood flow through the acoustic mechanism.

(2) Atherosclerosis. Narrowing large or small arteries may also include changes which conceivably may affect the acoustic mechanism.

(3) Capillary disease may result in interference in capillary exchange of nutrients and removal of waste substances through the capillary walls; this could affect hearing.

(4) The combination of segmental (patchy) arteriosclerosis of the medium-sized arteries plus capillary or arteriolar sclerosis may also tend to reduce the function of the acoustic mechanism.

industry and hearing

Fox, Meyer S. *"Medical Aspects of the Industrial Noise Problem,"* Industrial Medicine, 39: 19–22 (No. 6), June 1970.

A physician of Milwaukee, Wisconsin observes that noise exposure standards were established by the U.S. Department of Labor in 1969 and industrial failure to comply with these standards can lead to cancellation of government contracts with the company involved.

Occupational hearing loss is a hearing impairment that may have been caused by accidental injury or noise. Noise-induced hearing loss is that which occurs over a period of months or years of hazardous noise exposure and which involves a permanent, cumulative damage to nerve tissue involved in hearing.

Dr. Fox observes that statements have been made that noise will cause high blood pressure, circulatory and nervous disease, ulcers, stress reactions and so forth. He believes, however, that valid evidence of these relationships is lacking and that the only definite proof that we have is that noise can cause a hearing loss. The hearing loss may be temporary or permanent.

Noise can have non-auditory effects such as interference with speech and communication. Many noises which are not intense enough to injure hearing can interfere seriously with speech communication, which is important in employee training and performance.

industrial noise and hearing loss

J. Coleman Scal, "Hearing Impairment in Noisy Environment," New York State Journal of Medicine, 56: 2839–45 (No. 18), September 15, 1956.

J. Coleman Scal, M.D., of New York City, observes that industrial noise hazards capable of causing deafness have recently been brought to the attention of labor, industry, and insurance carriers.

Noise deafness develops very slowly and insidiously, and the worker in a noisy environment of 90 decibels or over is usually unaware of the danger and is apt to disregard his early symptoms. The early stage of noise deafness is usually characterized by the onset of tinnitus (ringing in the ears) which may or may not disappear after work stoppage or over the weekend. At this stage the worker experiences no difficulty in hearing, but if an audiogram is made at this time, it may show a loss in hearing at the 4,000 frequency mark. Thus, at the beginning of the exposure the low or speech range sounds have not been affected, and the worker has no difficulty in ordinary conversation.

Continued exposure to noise will further affect the frequencies around the 4,000 cycle, and hearing of the high or musical tones will become affected so that the worker will complain that he cannot hear the doorbell and telephone ring. This is a diagnostic sign in early perceptive deafness.

Most workers at one time or another are exposed to considerable noise during everyday activity without ill effects. We know that an average office shows a 30-decibel noise level, a busy street a 68-decibel noise level, heavy street traffic an 84-decibel noise level, and the subway an 85- to 90-decibel noise level. It is only when one works in an environment well above the everyday noise level that nerve deafness sets in.

The first symptoms a worker suffers after he starts to work in a noisy environment are tinnitus and a temporary loss in hearing which will disappear completely within a few hours after he leaves the noisy area. This is known as nerve fatigue and is considered by some hearing specialists as a metabolic process which stimulates and causes a disturbance of the hair cells of the cochlea. Early recognition of this condition and the beginning of suitable preventive measures may stop permanent hearing loss.

Dr. Scal reports six case histories in which nerve deafness occurred due to high noise levels.

It can be expected that if the worker continues in the noisy environment, additional hearing loss will develop. If he is removed from the noise, hearing loss will cease and some improvement may take place. The hearing loss can be considered permanent if there is no improvement after six months of complete removal from the noisy environment.

ultrasonics and progressive deafness

Angeluscheff, Zhivko D. "Ultrasonics and Progressive Deafness," Acta Oto-Laryngologica, 45: 7–13 (Fasc. 1), January–February 1955.

Zhivko D. Angeluscheff, of New York City and the Manhattan Eye, Ear and Throat Hospital, reports that the mechanized life of modern man is steadily exposing an increasing number of persons to hazards of hearing from sonic-ultrasonic impacts.

Pilots, forge workers, railroad employees, mechanics, and shipyard workers are suffering impairment of hearing in ever-rising numbers.

Any vibratory device emitting fast waves, being sensed as sound (sonic) or not (ultrasonic), above a specific range is capable of provoking functional structural changes in the hearing organ. If such exposure is long enough, the effect may result in damage of irreversible nature.

The exposure of the ear of experimental animals to low ultrasonics of 38,000 cycles per second for a period of seven days for 30 minutes daily has resulted in disastrous effects upon the hearing apparatus. When examined under the microscope no changes in the drum membrane and middle ear have been observed, but changes were found in the labyrinth and the inner ear. In the organ of Corti a disruption of the cell structures was found. The plasma of the hair cells was cloudy and the pillar cells were broken. Hemorrhages were found in the scala tympani, and especially about the round window and the cochlea. The hemorrhages originated in the capillaries of the endosteal lining of the scala tympani. The nerve and ganglionic cells were found to be shrunken and the fibers distorted. It was judged that the pathological damage and alteration of the lower turn of the cochlea was responsible for disappearance of perception of high-pitched tones. The bone and collagen of the ear responded late and slowly to injury. New bony tissue was found to penetrate the structure and cause fixation of the stapes and to thus initiate a progressive failing of the hearing.

Formation of new bony tissue at the oval window in the middle ear was judged to be the main pathological feature of otosclerosis.

20

drugs, allergies and injuries

Hearing can be affected adversely by a variety of damaging influences. Almost any drug may cause a loss of hearing if it has a predilection for the auditory nerve or associated structures. Certain antibiotics, for example, when taken internally may cause total deafness. Other drugs may reduce hearing acuity because of individual sensitivities to them.

Head injuries may cause a loss of hearing, as may direct damage to the hearing mechanism such as in a broken eardrum. The causes of some disorders of hearing have not been clearly established.

drugs and loss of hearing

Berk, Dennis P. and Thomas Chalmers. "Deafness Complicating Antibiotic Therapy of Hepatic Encephalopathy," Annals of Internal Medicine, 73: 393–96 (No. 3), September 1970.

Two physicians of Tufts University Medical School in Boston observe that the danger of hearing loss from the use of neomycin when taken internally is often overlooked.

The two physicians have seen five cases of deafness in a single hospital in patients whose illnesses were being treated with oral neomycin for liver disease. In one patient the deafness had its onset after about 10 months of daily intake of neomycin. She had almost total loss of hearing in one ear and severe impairment in the other. Another patient had the same antibiotic and after about two years she noticed her loss of hearing. She was shifted from neomycin to another antibiotic (paromomycin), but gradually lost her hearing until she could no longer hear normal conversation and hearing tests showed she had lost 20 decibels of hearing. Another patient suffered from 40 to 60 decibels loss in hearing within a short time and gradually became deaf. A fourth patient had suffered a sudden hearing loss in her left ear amounting to 50 to 60 decibels, with normal hearing in her right ear 27 years prior to hospital admission for liver disease. Her liver disease improved on treatment with neomycin and other care and she was discharged from the hospital with instructions to take small doses of neomycin and paromomycin. After about two months she noticed a loss of hearing in her right ear (the normal one). A few months later tests showed she was totally deaf in her left ear and had a loss of 40 to 60 decibels in the right ear. The fifth patient was treated with both neomycin and paromomycin and suffered a loss of hearing in both ears of 50 to 70 decibels.

The physicians examined the medical literature and found other reports of impairment of hearing after treatment internally with neomycin. The hearing loss appears to be permanent. Damage apparently is done to the hair cells of the internal ear.

Ordinarily neomycin is excreted by the kidneys and damage to hearing appears to be more severe when damage to the kidneys impairs their ability to excrete the drug. Paromomycin, according to the two physicians, has a chemical structure and toxic effects on the hearing mechanism that is quite close to that of neomycin and may have contributed to the hearing losses of two of the patients described above. Substitutes for the antibiotics described for the conditions treated have not yet been completely established by the medical profession.

deafness from allergy

Jordan, Raymond E. "Deafness Due to Allergy," Laryngoscope, 60: 152–60 (No. 2), February 1950.

Raymond E. Jordan, M.D., of Pittsburgh, discusses allergy as a factor in deafness. It is Dr. Jordan's conviction that allergy plays an important role, either as a cause or as a contributing factor, in many cases of deafness.

In a review of 110 cases of loss of hearing, Dr. Jordan found evidence that allergy of the middle or inner ear does exist and that it accounts for a high percentage of cases of deafness. Early diagnosis and treatment on an allergic basis has resulted in restoration of hearing in some cases.

allergy as a cause of fluid in the middle ear

Robert E. Boswell, "Allergies as Causes of Middle Ear Effusion," Ohio State Medical Journal, 52: 374 (No. 4), April 1956.

Robert E. Boswell, M.D., of the Miami Valley Hospital and the Good Samaritan Hospital in Dayton, Ohio, observes that fluid in the middle ear may originate in the blood serum, sometimes as a result of negative pressure alone and sometimes due to the added influence of an inflammation and increased capillary permeability. A primary cause of fluid in the middle ear, however, is an obstructed Eustachian tube, and it is probable that allergic phenomena account for about 15 per cent of such obstructions.

Whether the initial allergen be house dust, shellfish, sunlight, or emotional stress, the stimuli follow the same pathways and produce the same result, which is the accumulation of fluid and resultant tissue anoxia. The primary reaction begins in the blood vessels with dilatation of the small vessels. This, together with the increased permeability of the capillary walls, permits the loss of serum and electrolytes into the surrounding tissues, causing edema. It is the edema which produces the allergic manifestations. Continuous emotional stress may raise the sensitivity level of our psychosomatic mechanism. Patients laboring under unusual fear or anxiety suddenly become allergic to various stimuli to which they normally remain unresponsive.

ménière's disease

Williams, Henry L. "The Present Status of the Diagnosis and Treatment of Endolymphatic Hydrops (Ménière's Disease)." The Annals of Otology, Rhinology and Laryngology, 56: 614–46 (No. 3), September 1947.

Henry L. Williams, M.D., of Rochester, Minnesota, says that in 1861, Ménière described a disease of sudden attacks of nausea and vomiting with progressive deafness and pounding sound in the affected ear. He described in detail most of the characteristic symptoms and signs of the malady that came to be called by his name.

Dr. Williams further stated that the impairment of hearing might progress to complete deafness without any gross pathologic findings suggestive of disease in the ear.

The types of dizziness arising from the Ménière kind of ear disease are: 1) typical attacks in which the patient has the feeling that objects are rotating around him or that he himself is rotating; 2) a sensation of being forced to one side or the other, which sensation may be actually accompanied by an inability to walk straight; 3) attacks in which the patient is suddenly thrown to the ground either forward or backward as if he had been hit on the head with a hammer, and 4) occurrence of a more or less constant unsteadiness so that the patient has to hold onto a support and both feels and is unsteady.

Vertigo in the strict sense is an experience in which the patient has the sensation that the outer world is moving about him or that he himself is whirling in space. Frequently, however, the term vertigo is used erroneously as a synonym for dizziness or giddiness to indicate a disturbed relationship to surrounding objects in space. The terms "dizziness" and "giddiness" should be restricted to an abnormal sensation of unsteadiness characterized by a feeling of movement within the head, without the sensation of the external world or the patient himself being in motion.

Dr. Williams believes that the basic cause of Ménière's Disease is a physical allergy which brings about a reaction and the accumulation of excess fluid in the portion of the ear which is affected, by means of the parasympathetic nervous system. Although this hypothesis has not been definitely proved there is some evidence which supports this theory. The microscope, for example, reveals changes in the tissues of the ear which are found in allergy.

loss of hearing from head injury

Does, I. E. A. and T. Bottema. "Postraumatic Conductive Hearing Loss," Archives of Otolaryngology, 82: 331–39 (No. 4), October 1965.

Two physicians of the University of Utrecht in the Netherlands report a study of 15 persons who had impaired hearing as a result of injury to the head. The increasing frequency of traffic accidents, in which head injuries may occur, is cited as a matter of importance by the Dutch physicians in respect to the loss of hearing.

So far as hearing is concerned, an injury in which the temple is fractured is most important, because fractures of the petrosal bone (side of the head above the cheek bone) are apt to damage the middle ear, while the deeper or inner ear parts are left intact. A fracture in the side of the head (temporal area) may cause a rupture of the eardrum and facial nerve paralysis or a hemorrhage into the area of the eardrum.

Loss of hearing due to hemorrhage or rupture of the eardrum is apt to disappear within weeks, but in some patients a conductive hearing loss is apt to persist after all other healing. This study is concerned with 15 cases in which the hearing loss persisted after head injury.

Of the three small bones of the middle ear, which transmit sound vibrations from the eardrum to the deeper parts of the ear, the incus bone is most loosely supported and is predisposed to dislocation.

In this study surgical exploration through the eardrum in 13 of the 15 persons with loss of hearing following head injury revealed that the incus had been damaged or dislocated in 12 of the 13 surgical cases. Audiometric tests, x-rays of the middle ear, examination of the eardrum, a good history of the head injury, with or without bleeding from the ear, are not dependable in the diagnosis of this kind of injury. Only surgical exploration through the eardrum is able to provide the true explanation of the loss of hearing.

A 14-year-old schoolboy fell on his head during exercises on the horizontal bar. He suffered concussion and bleeding from the left ear. His hearing was lost on the left side. On exploratory surgery through the eardrum the bones of the middle ear were found to have been damaged. Placement of a pellet of connective tissue between the bones of the middle ear and the footplate improved hearing. A 15-year-old schoolgirl was involved in a traffic accident. She suffered a fractured skull, bleeding from the left ear, and a hearing loss on the left side. The eardrum appeared normal, but surgery revealed upward displacement of the incus. Hearing was improved following correction by surgery.

In only one patient of 13 surgical corrections was there a loss of hearing after surgery. It appears that surgical exploration and correction should be done when a person has a persistent hearing loss after head injury, especially if it involves the side of the head.

broken eardrums in children

Spector, Martin. "Tympanic Membrane Perforations in Children," Clinical Pediatrics, 3: 25–27 (No. 1), January 1964.

An ear specialist from the Temple Medical School of Philadelphia observes that broken eardrums are caused by injury or infection. In children the chief cause is an infection of the middle ear (otitis media). Less often, an injury to the ear from a direct blow, blast, concussion or head injury may cause the rupture. External ear infections rarely cause a perforation. Occasionally a small tumor of cholesterol and fat may be the source of a perforation.

The majority of broken eardrums tend to heal spontaneously, but chronic perforations lead to trouble in two ways: repeated infections of the ear and loss of hearing.

Surgical correction of a ruptured eardrum should be sought if the perforation has persisted for three to six months after all infection has been cleared from the ear, or if there has been a loss of hearing. If infections occur because water gets into the middle ear surgery should be done also.

Surgery should not be done if an infection cannot be cleared up, if there is a blocked Eustachian tube, or if a tumor cannot be completely removed. If an infection or tumor is buried under the surgeon's graft the troubles of the patient are aggravated rather than alleviated. If the Eustachian tube is blocked, closure of the broken eardrum results in persistent, serious infection of the middle ear (otitis media).

Vein tissue is a satisfactory grafting material at all ages for the closing of the space of a ruptured eardrum, but Fascia is an even more useful repair tissue and can be secured in quantities great enough to close even a massive perforation.

The invention of the operating binocular microscope (which provides binocular vision, magnifies six to 16 times, and gives ample light) has been a boon to all otologists (ear specialists). Other advances have also helped.

After the eardrum has been grafted the patient may leave the hospital in a day or two, but should be seen weekly since some discharge or secretion may need to be removed by the doctor. The graft surface is not cleared for three weeks because of the hazard of removal. There is

relatively little discomfort in this kind of surgery and the graft is successful
in about 90 per cent of the cases.

head injuries and inner ear damage

*Davey, Lycurgus M. "Labyrinthine Trauma in Head Injury," Connecticut
Medicine, 29: 250–53 (No. 4), April 1965.*

A surgeon of the Yale University School of Medicine reports that head injuries may result in damage to the labyrinth of the ear. The head injury
may be relatively slight, often insufficient to cause a loss of consciousness.

Dr. Davey analyzed 101 cases of head injuries in which there was some
damage to the ear. Fifty-seven of the 101 cases of dizziness following head
injuries were diagnosed as labyrinthine concussion.

The acute phase of this kind of injury usually lasts no more than 48
hours and is characterized by extreme vertigo in certain positions. Nausea
and vomiting may occur in certain positions. Recovery begins about the
third day and lasts for about two weeks. A convalescent stage may last for
as long as six months and may include some psychogenic reactions. A
chronic stage may last for 18–24 months but true vertigo will not be observed in this phase. Psychogenic factors may confuse the picture and
cause persons in this chronic phase to be labeled as psychoneurotics. Although loss of hearing may occur this is not discussed to any extent. Dr.
Davey believes the key to the evaluation of symptoms associated with injuries to the vestibular system of the ear lies in the understanding of the
complaint of dizziness.

21

hearing tests

The evolution of modern instruments for testing hearing and the establishment of standards for normal and impaired hearing is relatively recent.
Pure tone audiometry, speech audiometry, psychogalvanic skin testing and
other techniques for the measurement of hearing are now in existence for
individual or group testing. Even computer-averaging of electroencephalographic responses to sound has been used in diagnosis of deafness in infants. All, however, may involve errors in evaluation of hearing deficiencies and even hearing standards have been challenged as being unrealistic.
Nevertheless, the early detection of hearing defects facilitates diagnosis
and treatment and has become essential particularly in children and young
adults. In both group screening and individual exploration of the capacity
to hear the present hearing tests are invaluable.

hearing tests

*Guild, Stacy R. "Interpretation of Hearing Tests," Journal of the Ameri-
can Medical Association, 142: 466–69 (No. 7), February 18, 1950.*

Stacy R. Guild, Ph.D., of Baltimore, says that nothing is gained clinically
by making hearing tests that cannot be interpreted with reasonable certainty in terms of cause.

No microscopic evidence exists to support or to refute the diagnostic
interpretations customarily made of data obtained by most of the elaborate, time-consuming techniques that have been devised and advocated in
recent years for testing various aspects of the hearing function.

Often a so-called diagnosis is in reality only a description of the kinds
of hearing defects found by the tests made. The clinical history and the
physical examination are of great importance in the interpretation of hearing tests, either in terms of damage responsible for the impaired function
or in terms of treatment.

For most patients a few simple tests of hearing afford all the information the ear specialist needs to supplement or to confirm the impressions

gained from the history and the physical examination. A clear distinction should be made between tests for research purposes and tests for clinical purposes.

evolution of hearing tests

Goetzinger, C. P. "Hearing Tests," Journal of the Kansas Medical Society, 58: 94–95 (No. 2), February 1957.

C. P. Goetzinger, Ph.D., of the University of Kansas School of Medicine, reports that the accurate measurement of hearing did not become a reality until the invention of the vacuum-tube pure-tone audiometer.

Although the electronic pure-tone audiometer appeared in this country in 1921, it was not until 1939 that adequate norms had been established to evaluate average normal hearing. Since that time the pure-tone audiometer has been shown to be an exceedingly useful means for the appraisal of hearing acuity.

During World War II it became necessary to study the transmission and reception of signals under heavy noise conditions. Thousands of English words were studied with reference to intelligibility, carrying power, and so on. As a result of this work, speech tests were developed which subsequently proved effective in the evaluation of hearing loss. In brief, it became possible to measure directly not only auditory acuity for speech but also how well the elements of speech could be understood. Hence, tests were provided for measuring hearing in the practical dimension of utilizing the elements of language, or words.

The advent of speech audiometry, or testing with words, has in no way detracted from the pure tone audiometric test. When one is used in conjunction with the other, a more complete picture of a person's ability to hear is available.

In the above tests of hearing, a response is required of the person. In other words, he is expected to raise his finger, press a button, or repeat a word, depending upon the nature of the signal. Many ingenious methods, such as the Peep Show, have been worked out to elicit responses from children. With infants and very young children who are unable to respond in an appropriate manner, attention has been focused on a change of behavior in response to sound.

The search for a method to measure thresholds for hearing objectively has resulted in the development of psychogalvanic skin audiometry. In short, auditory sensitivity is determined by a decrease in the electrical resistance of the skin when a tone is sounded. Two electrodes, connected to appropriate recording equipment, are placed on certain parts of the body. A mild electric shock capable of evoking a decrease in skin resistance is paired with a pure tone, until the tone by itself initiates the desired response.

Further research is needed on the psychogalvanic skin-testing technique before it can be used clinically on a wide-spread scale for the measurement of hearing acuity.

three screening methods for detection
of hearing loss

Yankauer, Alfred, Margaret L. Geyer, and Helen C. Chase. "Comparative Evaluation of Three Screening Methods for Detection of Hearing Loss in School Children," American Journal of Public Health, 44: 77–82 (No. 1), January 1954.

Yankauer, Geyer, and Chase report a study involving a comparison of three different types of screening for hearing losses of school children.

Most workers in the field of audiology have stated for some time that individual pure-tone sweep check screening identifies more children with hearing loss for speech perception, as well as for tones above speech range, than group voice testing with fading numbers.

This study consisted of a comparative evaluation of screening for hearing loss by the individual sweep check, the "old" Massachusetts hearing test, and the group voice fading-numbers test. Nine public schools in Rochester, New York, were selected for the study. The study group was composed of 2,404 pupils. The screening procedures, diagnostic tests, and otologic appraisals were carried out within a period of two to three weeks for each of the nine school groups. The tests were performed in classrooms or other schoolrooms selected for low noise levels.

All of the 2,404 children received three screening tests: group phonograph, group pure tone, and individual sweep check.

As a result of this screening combination it was found that 118 children, or approximately 5 per cent of the total group, had a verified hearing loss.

No one of the three screening procedures was able to select all of the 118 children with hearing defects. The group phonograph screening procedure detected 33 per cent of the hard-of-hearing children, the group pure-tone screening test found 69 per cent of those with hearing losses, and the individual sweep check screening found 95 per cent of the children with hearing losses.

All of the children with verified hearing loss were seen by an otologist.

Educational recommendations, varying from preferred seating arrangements to speech reading instructions, were the joint decision of otologist and audiologist. Of the 118 children with verified hearing loss, medical or educational recommendations were made in 64 per cent of the cases. In the remaining children the verified hearing loss was of such a nature as not to require medical or educational attention at the time of examination.

Although the individual sweep check was the best case-finder of the three screening procedures, it selected more children with no hearing loss than either of the other two tests. This overselection, however, was not significantly in excess of the number of children overselected by either of the group tests.

It was found in this study that pure-tone techniques were significantly better screening devices than the group fading-numbers test. Of the two pure-tone techniques, the sweep check was the better case finder, but it required more than twice as much time to perform.

are hearing standards realistic?

House, Howard P. "Hearing Standards—Fact or Fiction?" Archives of Otolaryngology, 90: 208–13 (No. 2), August 1969.

A physician of the Otologic Medical Group of Los Angeles raises the question as to whether or not school placement standards for pupils are realistic in respect to their levels of hearing.

His interest in this subject developed because of the disappointment of parents of children with hearing handicaps and their despair due to unrealistic school placement hearing standards. Dr. House observes that many times children with impaired hearing are placed in various school programs on the basis of audiograms rather than the child's ability to perform in his environment. The child's entire future may be altered by a decision that places him in a different educational environment.

Too often, Dr. House believes, a child who is pronounced "profoundly deaf" may function well with a hearing aid in a school program for the hard of hearing. He also believes that the so-called hard of hearing child who may be assigned to an integrated hard-of-hearing program may be able to function as a normal-hearing child if adequate use is made of his residual hearing with a hearing aid. The following cases in Dr. House's practice illustrate the foregoing points.

A nine-year-old child had a hearing impairment due to German measles of the mother during pregnancy. A hearing aid had been used since the age of two. In school at the age of six the child functioned well and received grades of mostly A and B. After an audiogram the parents were told the child had been classified as profoundly deaf and must attend a school for the deaf. After one semester in the school for the deaf, the child lost all interest and motivation and his language and speech deteriorated considerably. After considerable difficulty this boy was returned to an integrated hard-of-hearing program and is again performing well.

Hearing loss in a two-year-old girl was diagnosed and a hearing aid was obtained immediately. A twin brother helped with a constant flow of communication. The parents worked diligently in auditory and speech reading before she was three years of age. The child graduated from a large suburban high school with better than average grades. Fortunately, she was never placed in a deaf school on the basis of her audiogram.

Dr. House reports other examples of unrealistic classifications of school children on the basis of audiograms and urges that a close look must be taken at the child rather than the audiogram. If he functions well in his environment with good intelligence, good vision, and with hearing aids, he may be able to function well as a "hard-of-hearing" child rather than a deaf one. Other children may be able to function as essentially normal hearing children in spite of a "hard-of-hearing" audiogram. The future of these children lies in the intelligence of those responsible for their placement, according to Dr. House.

errors in the diagnosis of hearing deficiency

Rosenberg, Philip E. "Misdiagnosis of Children with Auditory Problems," Journal of Speech and Hearing Disorders, 31: 279–83 (No. 3), August 1966.

A hearing specialist from the Temple University School of Medicine in Philadelphia reports that occasionally in the diagnosis of children with hearing problems, certain incorrect labels ("auditory scramble," "nerve deafness"), which imply central hearing loss, are attached.

A large number of children who had been diagnosed as having central hearing loss were examined at the Audiology Department of Temple University Medical Center. The children had a characteristic history. In most cases, the parents were aware of the problem when the child was very young. Medical consultation was obtained at approximately one year of age. The parents were then referred to an audiologist or to a speech and hearing clinic. After a period of testing, the child was found to have hearing impairment, and a diagnosis of one of the types of central hearing loss was made.

Many of the children were placed in educational situations designed specifically for children with central hearing loss. Frequently the educational attempts resulted in failure and another round of examinations began. It was at this point that the author and his colleagues saw most of the children.

It was found that the majority of these children had peripheral (outer), not central, hearing impairment. Confused or incorrect early diagnosis had led to severe educational problems for many of these children. Some had been placed in educational surroundings completely unsuitable for them.

Although it is sometimes difficult to test the hearing of a very young child, certain suitable techniques, both old and new, are available. Some of the newer methods include a technique whereby an electrode is placed in a part of the ear and nerve action potential from the living ear is picked up and recorded. There are also new types of x-ray studies far superior to the old for detecting auditory defects. All test results should be interpreted by standard scientific methodology. Casual immediate reading and interpretation of test results may be extremely misleading.

Many of the children tested by the authors were found to have essentially normal hearing in the lowest frequencies. They responded to low voices and gross noisemakers. Nevertheless, their auditory deficits were still severe. If the specific type of hearing loss can be determined accurately at a young age, suitable remedial steps may be taken. Expert and appropriate teaching by a trained specialist may well result in a dramatic and exciting improvement in the child's speech and language development.

exposing malingering of deafness

Pratt, Loring W. "Malingering of Deafness," Journal of the Maine Medical Association, 46: 43–45 (No. 2), February 1955.

Loring W. Pratt, M.D., of Waterville, Maine, reports that there are several ways in which the malingerer of deafness can be exposed.

Hearing tests of a suspected malingerer should be made only in the presence of a third party, who understands the testing procedure and who can be utilized as a witness if the subject makes some response which would be inappropriate in a deaf person.

The methods for exposing the malingerer of deafness are as follows:

1 *Psychological trickery.* In this type of exposure the patient is led to believe that something is true and when he acts upon this belief he is exposed. For example, the classic trick is for the examiner to drop a silver dollar behind the patient at the close of the examination. If he immediately turns, picks it up, and passes it to the physician, he is exposed. None but an extremely naive malingerer could be exposed by this procedure.

2 *Reading test.* When a normal individual is given material to read, and a masking tone is gradually increased in his ear, his voice will gradually increase in intensity so that he may hear what he is saying over the level of the masking tone. If a truly deaf person is given such reading to do, a masking tone does not affect the intensity of his reading voice. If one who claims to suffer from bilateral deafness is given such a reading test, and his voice intensity increases with the increasing level of the masking tone, he is established as being able to hear.

3 *Speech feedback.* This is a new technique by which reading material is given to the subject. He reads it while wearing a headset through which delicate electronic devices return his speech to his ears a few hundredths of a second later than he would ordinarily hear it. This abnormal feedback causes him to stutter. Of course, if he were truly deaf, this sort of apparatus would have no effect at all on his ability to read without stuttering.

4 *Physiologic testing.* These tests are often utilized in determining the ability of tiny children to hear sound, before the age of the patient permits accurate testing. They are easily applied to suspected malingerers of total deafness. Although they provide the physician with useful information about the patient, these tests by themselves do not produce adequate legal evidence of malingering.

If a loud noise is suddenly produced behind the unsuspecting patient, he will blink, reflexly. No such response is found in the deaf.

A sudden loud noise produced behind the unsuspecting patient produces an immediate constriction of the pupils followed by their dilatation. This test, as in the previous example, is not admissible as evidence in court, but it often provides the physician a lead as to the validity of the claim of total deafness.

5 *Psychogalvanic testing.* It has been shown by a number of authors that it is possible to test hearing by means of a measurement of changes in the electrical resistance of the skin of the hand or arm. The subject is made to develop a conditioned reflex and then responds reflexly to stimuli when presented. This is often used to test the hearing of young children who are unable to co-operate with audiometry. This "lie-detector" sort of test provides us with a good deal of information, but evidence from it is inadmissible in court.

The foregoing tests are designed to expose the patient who claims deafness in both ears. The patient who claims to be deaf in one ear may be exposed by the following tests if he is a malingerer:

1 *Repetition test.* In this technique, the subject is fitted to a headset from which connections are so arranged that speech directed into a microphone may be shifted from ear to ear without his awareness of the act. Then he is told a story which has been formulated so that certain details are heard by his good ear but certain other details are heard in only the supposed deaf ear. He is then asked to repeat the story, going into as much detail as possible. He need repeat only one detail spoken into the "deaf" ear to expose himself as a malingerer.

2 *Stenger test.* This test relies upon the fact that normal hearing is dependent upon the quantity of the masking tone present at the time of the test. A simple test may be done with two 512-cycle tuning forks. One fork should be given a standard stimulation, and the distance at which it can be heard by the good ear should be recorded. Then this test should be repeated while a similarly stimulated fork is held at one-fourth this distance from the alleged deaf ear. If the fork is heard at the same point on this occasion, the patient is deaf; but if it is necessary to move the fork closer to his head than was necessary without the masking tone, he is not deaf.

A modification of this test may be performed by slipping a rubber tube over the stem of the tuning fork. The end of this tube is then held at the external ear. If this masking tone produces change in the distance the testing fork must be held from the head, the subject is not deaf.

the computer and the EEG in testing
hearing of infants

Barnet, Ann B. and Ann Lodge. "Diagnosis of deafness in infants with the use of computer-averaged electroencephalographic responses to sound," Journal of Pediatrics, 69: 753–58 (No. 5), November 1966.

Two members of the Washington School of Psychiatry and the Children's Hospital of the District of Columbia say that most hearing specialists would agree that special training of the deaf infant should be started well before the second birthday to minimize risks of impairment in language development.

Hearing losses in young children are difficult to ascertain and it is not always possible to determine how much of a handicap the child has, especially if he has other sensory or motor handicaps or developmental retardation.

In this research 22 infants were tested and 12 were found to have decreased responses to sound as measured by the electroencephalogram. Although the study was restricted to babies whose hearing might have been affected by German measles, the authors concluded that EEG audiometry may be a useful tool for discovering hearing losses in young children regardless of the causes.

auditory screening of infants

Caziarc, Donald R. "Auditory Screening of Infants," California's Health. 20: 129 (No. 17), March 1, 1963.

A hearing conservation specialist of the California State Department of Health reviews the problem of detecting hearing losses in infants and reports that modern research has resulted in the production of a screening procedure that has been standardized for infants of eight months of age.

The test consists of a few sounds presented at a level of approximately 40 decibels and includes a soft, pleasant voice for the low frequencies, a middle-range rattle for the frequencies essential to speech and unvoiced consonants, s-s-s and k-k-k representing the higher frequencies. The intensity of the sounds is controlled by the examiner at a prescribed distance from the child's ear.

A study in Baltimore of more than 700 children who "failed" an auditory screening test suggests that 60 per cent of such children have significant psychological problems and that 34 per cent have abnormalities of the nervous system. Thus, failure to pass a simplified auditory screening test may suggest the need for more intensive examinations.

22

treatment of hearing losses

Treatment of hearing losses may involve the psychological and work readjustment of the individual. Sometimes treatment can be successful in restoration of hearing, while at other times no effective treatment is available. Modern surgery has made considerable progress in the treatment of hearing deficiencies, but some losses are beyond any medical or surgical efforts at restoration.

Hearing aids and speech reading are not universal solutions to hearing losses. Nevertheless, modern medical treatment is sometimes highly successful and can usually help to improve hearing or to retard further loss.

adjustments of the hard-of-hearing

Adams, Eris L. "Adjustment of the Hard of Hearing After Leaving the Service," United States Naval Medical Bulletin, Supplement, 46: 249–52, March 1946.

Eris L. Adams, United States Naval Reserve, reports a follow-up study of 504 hard-of-hearing veterans who received training and equipment to overcome their handicap at the Hearing and Speech Rehabilitation Unit of the Philadelphia Naval Hospital. The study was based on a questionnaire mailed to 1,272 former patients. Full data were secured from 504 of the returns.

The following information was gained from the study:

(1) Ninety-four per cent of the men were still using their hearing aids.

(2) Sixty-six per cent reported their hearing acuity had remained the same as at the time of discharge.

(3) Twenty-four per cent had difficulty in obtaining batteries for their hearing aids.

(4) Eight per cent had been unable to get repair service for the hearing aid. This figure is probably low because few repairs would have been

needed during the two-month interval between discharge and the time of answering the questionnaire.

(5)   Twenty-three per cent had been refused a job or had been unsuccessful on a job because of hearing deficiency.

(6)   Fifty-two per cent reported that lip reading had helped them "greatly"; 35 per cent had been hleped "moderately," and 13 per cent "slightly."

(7)   Forty-five per cent of the patients had continued lip-reading studies since discharge.

The major problems of adjustment as indicated by this study of hard-of-hearing patients fell into four categories: 1) care of residual hearing; 2) maintenance of maximum mechanical performance of the hearing aid; 3) adjustment to the job in terms of the hearing loss, and 4) achievement of the relatively proper mental-hygiene level in relation to the social and economic processes.

lip reading

Pauls, Miriam D., Harriet L. Haskins, and William G. Hardy. VIII. Speech Reading, Auditory Training and Speech Correction in the Re-education Program," United States Naval Medical Bulletin, Supplement, 46: 232–38, March 1946.

Miriam D. Pauls, Harriet L. Haskins, and William G. Hardy, of the United States Navy, say that speech reading (sometimes called lip reading) is a complex process. Every conversational situation includes many factors beyond the speech reader's control. Moreover, the conversation may be complicated by poor speech, poor lighting, and general confusion, with the result that even the most expert speech reader is at a disadvantage.

Ideas presented must be grasped in a fleeting instant. Only about a third of speech movements are visible and the whole process is an ever-changing continuum. To these variables must be added the facts that no two mouths are alike, nor are there two people who talk in the same way.

In lip reading, patients are taught to feel, hear, and see simultaneously. They are taught to recognize some of the cues that are associated with a typical speech situation: gestures, facial expression, objects handled or referred to, the place and the personality of the speaker.

In the program of hearing and speech rehabilitation at the United States Naval Hospital in Philadelphia, the lip-reading patient has 20 basic lessons of an hour's duration, each supplemented by special classes to provide additional practice. Instruction is given in small groups of five to eight patients. Each classroom is equipped with a small sound-treated, well-lighted booth with a large glass partition that separates it from the rest of the room. This device provides valuable silent practice in which no auditory cues can be heard, and demonstrates that the student can follow a conversation without actually hearing the spoken words.

The speaker sits in the booth and talks in a normal conversational voice without exaggeration or distortion of the speech pattern. Characteristic gestures and facial expressions are freely employed.

After four weeks of training a proficiency test is given to each patient. The results of this test are used to plan further training for the patient.

Each lesson is organized around a central theme. This gives unity and point to the lesson and is an aid to the student in that he knows to some extent what to anticipate. In the basic series, everyday experiences determine the selected topics and are constructed around the hospital, a restaurant, a bank, shopping and so on. Topics selected for the more advanced groups depend upon special interests.

Skits are acted out by members of the group in order to develop powers of observation as well as to train the class to follow rapid dialogue. Other practice situations are also used, such as well-acted movie scenes.

At the time of this report 2,787 men had been given training in this Aural Rehabilitation Unit.

speech reading

Butler, Stahl. "Continuing Therapy for Hard-of-Hearing Patients," Journal of the Michigan State Medical Society, 55: 72 ff. (No. 1), January 1956.

Stahl Butler, Executive Director of the Michigan Association for Better Hearing at Lansing, says that many people have the mistaken notion that lip reading, or speech reading, is used only by the severely hard-of-hearing, or the deaf.

As a matter of fact, speech reading is a skill that can be used to great advantage by many people with normal hearing and it is the only non-medical assistance that is available for people with slight hearing losses where the use of a hearing aid is not justified.

Because the sounds that are the most difficult to hear are the easiest to see on the lips, a hearing aid and lip reading supplement each other perfectly and provide social adequacy, even for people with severe hearing losses. Though a hearing aid may help a person to hear much better, the hearing aid never provides normal hearing, and there is always the need to supplement the hearing aid with lip reading.

The shy, withdrawn patient, suffering from a psychological handicap because of his hearing deficiency, benefits greatly from the group aspects of a lip reading class.

In Michigan, speech correction instruction is available through the public schools in most of the major southern communities and to a limited extent in the northern part of the state.

hearing aids for children

Gaeth, John H. and Evan Lounsbury. "Hearing Aids and Children in Elementary Schools," Journal of Speech and Hearing Disorders. 31: 283–89 (No. 3), August 1966.

Two hearing specialists of Wayne State University report that there have been very few studies of the child in elementary school who wears a hearing aid. This report is based upon a study of 134 children in the Detroit area who had been provided hearing aids. Ages varied from three to 18.

Ten per cent of the parents who were interviewed reported that their children never wore their hearing aids, and only 32 per cent wore their aids at school, home, and play. Ninety per cent did wear the hearing aids at school and 55 per cent of this group wore the aid at home also. One child used his hearing aid at home, but never at school.

Academic progress could not be measured for all children because some were in preschool or kindergarten classes, rooms for the hard of hearing, or ungraded special education classes. Of 90 children, however, who did not fit into these categories, 50 per cent had failed one or more grades.

Analysis of the hearing aids revealed that 45 per cent had feedback problems, defective controls, cracked receivers, distorting or noisy amplifiers, or other defects. At best 55 per cent of the hearing aids could be considered adequate.

Only 16 per cent of the children met the original requirements of the investigators for adequate hearing-aid use. By more lenient standards no more than 50 per cent of the children were getting any benefit at all from their hearing aids.

The study also revealed that the parents knew very little about a hearing aid and its care, and misjudged the value of the hearing aid as well as its relationship to school progress. Routine orientation programs for the parents of children with hearing aids are needed, according to the two investigators.

effects of delayed treatment

Elliott, Lois L. and Ann B. Vegely. "Some Possible Effects of the Delay of Early Treatment of Deafness: A Second Look," Journal of Speech and Hearing Research, 11: 833–36 (No. 3), September 1968.

Two members of the Central Institute for the Deaf in St. Louis, Missouri reported a study of the effects of hearing losses in children in terms of education and learning.

The study was concerned with the age at which a hearing aid was first worn and age of first attendance at a school for the deaf as well as certain other information.

Data on 252 children in a state-supported school for the deaf were obtained. A group of hard-of-hearing children in a private school who first began wearing hearing aids at the age of three or less was compared with the state school pupils who did not begin wearing hearing aids until the age of five or six years. It was found that the children who were fitted with hearing aids at older ages showed lower achievement scores than children who were given hearing aids earlier.

surgical treatment

Work, Walter P. "Types of Hearing Losses Amenable to Surgical Treatment," Medical Center Journal, 32: 63-66 (No. 2), March-April 1966.

A physician of the Department of Otorhinolaryngology at the University of Michigan reports that within the last 30 years surgery for persons with conduction hearing losses has advanced rapidly. Surgery for the restoration of natural hearing has few complications and they occur in less than 4 per cent of the patients. Dr. Work discusses surgery for hearing losses due to otosclerosis, serous otitis media, congenital anomalies, injury, acute and chronic infections of the middle ear and Ménière's Disease.

The surgical treatment of otosclerosis involves the stapes, one of the three tiny bones that conduct sound waves across the middle ear. The surgeon can raise the tympanic membrane (eardrum) and examine the stapes footplate that blocks sound from the inner ear because of its invasion by the spongy bone disease that is known as otosclerosis. The surgeon may then remove the footplate and replace it with a combination of available substances that reestablishes a pathway for the sound waves. Vein grafts, plastic materials, wire and fat grafts, a wire and gelfoam, Teflon and other substances may be used. Many patients who were operated on 10 years ago can still hear.

Surgery for serous otitis media (fluid in the middle ear) is the most common cause of loss of hearing in children. Of 18,000 children with hearing losses in Michigan 80 per cent owed their affliction to fluid in the middle ear. Fortunately, if treated properly, most of these hearing losses can be permanently corrected. Surgical treatment is aimed at removal of fluid from the middle ear and correction of eustachian tube (channel from the throat to the middle ear) function. Removal of tonsils and adenoids may be helpful also. Some of the surgeon's work can be done in his office.

Surgery for congenital abnormalities involving the conduction hearing apparatus may involve the external ear as well as the middle ear. Surgery is usually done only if the defects present at birth involve the ears on both sides, for if one ear is sound hearing may be sufficient. If plastic surgery for the outer ear is needed it should be delayed until surgical correction of hearing is achieved. Surgery for correction of congenital defects that cause loss of hearing is difficult and may have to be done in stages.

Surgery for hearing losses due to head injuries such as fractures of the temporal bone, penetrating wounds from bullets or other objects, slaps or blows over the ear, atmosphere pressure or other injuries may require replacement of middle ear bones (ossicles), reconstruction of the auditory canal, extraction of objects from the external auditory canal, repair of the tympanic membrane (eardrum) and other procedures.

Surgery for acute and chronic middle ear infections (suppurative otitis media) requires perforation of the eardrum for removal of pus even when antibiotics are used, and this form of surgery should be done early. The perforations are repaired by the grafting of skin, veins, or fascia to the tympanic membrane (eardrum). The ossicles (bones) of the middle ear may have to be replaced or reconstructed. Other surgery may be needed.

Surgery for Ménière's disease, which is characterized by attacks of ringing in the ear, deafness, and dizziness (vertigo) may be designed to destroy the labyrinth. In this type of surgery balance and hearing functions are both destroyed in the operated ear; however, the surgery is not done on a person who has serviceable hearing in the ear. The surgery is done only on a patient who is incapacitated by his vertigo (dizziness) and who does not have hearing in the affected ear.

The newer techniques of surgery for patients with hearing losses have been made possible by magnification, improved instruments, new surgical techniques, improved lighting and suction, and to some extent by the use of antibiotic and sulfa drugs. Today, the average patient with a conduction hearing loss has an excellent chance that hearing can be improved or restored by surgery.

23

community relationships

Community programs for the conservation of hearing involve the services of many different professional persons, such as the otolaryngologist, the pediatrician, the audiometrist, the speech therapist, the social worker, the educator, the psychologist, the psychiatrist and still others. An effective hearing program is costly in the construction of needed facilities, the purchase of essential equipment, the employment of adequate personnel and use of professional consultants. The American Society for the Hard of Hearing is one of the organizations that has provided leadership in this field, along with schools, governmental agencies and other groups.

a five-year kansas project

Gendel, Evalyn S. "Hearing Conservation of Children—A Special Five-Year Project in Kansas," American Journal of Public Health, 58: 499–504 (No. 3), March 1968.

A medical member of the State Department of Health in Topeka, Kansas says that children with an undetected hearing loss have been described by parents and teachers as "stubborn, aggressive, withdrawn, retarded, delinquent, defiant." Such behaviors result in underachievement, dropping out of school, delinquency and alienation of children from their families.

Kansas studies of a county prison farm revealed that hearing loss and deafness figured high in the group of inmates. In reformitories for boys and girls in Kansas the percentages afflicted with hearing losses was approximately three to five times greater than the national average.

This particular report is concerned with an on-going five year project in Kansas in which detection of hearing loss and its early follow-up and treatment are being emphasized and demonstrated. At the time of this report 35,435 children had received a hearing screening test in 24 counties of Kansas. A mobile hearing testing unit manned by two audiologists and a public health nurse was used to provide modern equipment at school centers in the program. The screening revealed 1,404 children with hearing losses and these children were referred for medical follow-up.

Although specific causes of hearing losses were not identified, Dr. Gendel observes that in Kansas the number of children exposed early in life to gun blasts from hunting and to tractor noise is high. Many young children learn to hunt by the age of eight years and to drive tractors or accompany their fathers on them as early as 12 years of age.

The study is continuing as of the above date with diagnostic clinics being made available by ear-nose-and-throat specialists in private practice. No treatment is given in these clinics, but after diagnosis the family doctor may then carry on.

Numerous groups, agencies, and organizations are involved in the study. The Kansas City Association of Trusts and Foundations, the U.S. Public Health Service, the State Department of Health, the Kansas Medical Society, the State Department of Public Instruction, the University of Kansas Medical Center, school systems, and other individuals and organizations are examples of the groups involved.

a community program to provide hearing services

Wallace, Helen M., John F. Daly, Robert Hui, Margaret A. Losty, and Donald Markle, "Community Program to Provide Hearing Services," Journal of the American Medical Association, 162: 719-23 (No. 8), October 20, 1956.

Wallace, Daly, Hui, Losty, and Markle, of New York City, report that scientific and technical progress in the field of hearing has occurred so rapidly that a new field of study has resulted.

Although much can be accomplished by the individual otologist in uncomplicated hearing problems, there remain a large number of patients who require, not cne or two specialists, but many in order to reach the fullest degree of rehabilitation. The team approach has been the natural outgrowth of this need and will be the determining factor in the quality of patient care. The large number of patients requiring these services in the community and the cost of developing and operating such services have made this a responsibility of the community.

Over a period of three years, a series of steps were taken to develop new services and to strengthen existing ones for children and adults with hearing problems in New York City. These steps included the formation of an advisory committee of experts drawn from the fields of otolaryngology, pediatrics, audiology, speech therapy, social service, education, and vocational rehabilitation. A recommendation was made by the advisory committee that a number of hearing centers be developed in the larger general teaching hospitals in the community. The committee also recommended the establishment of standards for hopsital hearing centers, a survey of all known existing services in the community, assistance to interested hospitals for the development of hearing centers, payment for cost of services by official health agencies, and the strengthening of case finding in school children by the provision of additional, modern audiometric testing equipment for use by the local school system.

A survey of 24 agencies that provided services for patients with hearing problems was carried out in New York City for the purpose of determining what personnel, facilities, and programs could be considered adequate for a complete, integrated service.

It was found that for maximum usefulness, a rehabilitation center for the hard-of-hearing needs both medical supervision by otologists and pediatricians and associated skills supplied by such personnel as audiologists, speech therapists, nurses, social workers, and psychologists.

It was recommended from this survey that the physical facilities of the hearing center should include sound-treated areas for diagnosis and therapy, reception and observation rooms, ear mold and electronics laboratories and other areas that added up to about 2,500 square feet of floor space.

It was concluded that there are advantages in locating the hearing center in a hospital connected with a medical school.

It was also concluded that a hearing program is costly and that the general community must be prepared to assist in the financing of such a program. Financing the cost of construction, equipment and operation of hearing centers appears to constitute the crux in the initiation of a community hearing program and in the provision of a high quality of service in the care of patients. The cost of construction may be borne by the individual hospital, by private philanthropy, by the Hospital Survey and

Construction Act, by government (in the case of governmental hospitals), or by any combination thereof.

index

index